Best Diet Products

Table of Contents

Chapter 9: A Plan, A Path, A Promise, A New You! 187

Chapter 10: Keeping the Journey Alive200

Conclusion 207

Introduction

Thank you for purchasing "Best Diet Products"! By doing so, you've already taken a huge step towards a new, healthier lifestyle, and that's really exciting! This book is designed to help you navigate the often-overwhelming amount of available information about weight loss and get you started on a journey to meet your goals and be the best 'you' that you can be; in these pages, you'll find accessible, easy-to-read data and advice for crafting a weight loss plan that WORKS now to help you lose and later to help you maintain your goals. This isn't just a book about dieting; it's a book about taking a journey to change.

Everyone chooses to lose weight for deeply personal reasons, and with so many fads and diets out there, how can you know what's safe, effective, and viable for *you*? "Best Diet Products" aims to take you from Day One to Day Forever with valuable insight into pills and supplements, meal replacement options, nutritional guidance, exercises for both body and mind, and simple, healthful recipes. We're not going to tell you WHAT to do; we're going to make sure you know HOW and WHY different approaches to changing your diet will work and give you the tools to make informed, positive decisions for yourself.

The following chapters will explore the use of supplements and pills, both for adding nutritional value and curbing your food cravings. Supplements can be used to regulate your digestive system, provide your body with nutrients that may be lacking in your diet, and reduce your appetite to help you eat less. There are many varieties of both pharmaceutical and herbal supplements on the market today, so it's important to have solid information before choosing a regimen that's right for you.

You'll also learn about using smoothies and shakes as meal replacement options, which can save you calories each day, while still helping you feel full and satisfied. By teaching you about the types of shakes and shake mixes available, you'll be better prepared to decide if this is a good choice for your weight loss needs. By looking at how smoothies can be made at home from every-day, easy-to-obtain ingredients, you'll be given another fantastic alternative for a satisfying meal without a ton of empty calories.

Because sometimes it isn't what you eat, but when you eat, that limits your metabolism, "Diet Products" will also take a look at the inner workings of intermittent fasting. This method is used to jumpstart and 'train' your body into taking in and using calories at the right time for maximum effectiveness. In conjunction with other weight loss contributors, it can be a useful tool in learned and applied discipline to help you lose weight safely and efficiently.

"Best Diet Products" will also explore the relationship between consumption and metabolism by looking at the effects that stimulants like caffeine and sugar can have on the body. By being aware of some of the hidden side effects lurking in the products you use every day, you'll be able to make more healthful choices for yourself and your weight loss journey. And because no one likes to give up their morning jolt, you'll also learn about alternatives to excess caffeine and sugars to help get you moving and satisfy your sweet tooth without breaking the calorie bank.

In fact, "Best Diet Products" will also arm you with the information to read and understand any food label. By understanding the relationship between empty calories, useful calories, real food, and filler ingredients, you'll be able to make choices about what you consume and how it will affect your metabolism and weight. You'll also learn about portion sizes, and how to adjust your meals to get more filling, useful calories and dump the empty calories for good. Because foods aren't inherently good or bad, you'll learn how to moderate your intake for healthy results. You'll also get some fun, easy recipes that will make you think about new ways to use the ingredients you already have in your kitchen.

Moving through the book, you'll also find a chapter on getting you moving. One of the most limiting factors on any weight loss journey is the ability and the desire to exercise. That's because exercise sounds boring and difficult! But it doesn't have to be, because exercise doesn't always mean an expensive gym membership or running a marathon. Exercise can be anything that gets your blood pumping and you moving- and you'll learn how to get in your cardio and your weight training without ever setting foot inside a gym, unless you want to, of course!

Exercise isn't only good for the body; it's also good for the mind. A workout can make you feel good, raising endorphins along with your heart rate. Mental exercise can also help you lose weight by reducing the stress hormones that can cause you to overeat, overthink, and lose sleep! When you're stressed out, your metabolism can get off the rails, causing you to lose your appetite and then make up for it by binge-eating, or making you lack the sleep your body needs to heal, rest, and metabolize new cells. "Best Diet Products" will help you learn to manage stress and make thoughtful food and exercise choices through meditation and mindfulness techniques that anyone can use!

In the last chapters of the book, you'll discover ways to put together everything you've learned and craft a weight-loss plan that works for your lifestyle, your budget, and your available time commitments. That's right; it doesn't have to consume your entire day to lose weight! Who has time to work out for hours, slave over elaborate recipes, and still not feel well-fed or hard-working enough? Nobody, and you don't have to feel that way either. Small adjustments can effect big change, and if you want to lose weight safely, efficiently, and permanently, then creating a feasible plan is crucial to meeting your goals.

Before you get started on Chapter 1, take a moment to congratulate yourself for taking the leap and purchasing this book. Let this be the beginning of a beautiful relationship between you, your mental and physical health, your eating and exercise habits, and a brand new outlook on weight loss and real life. Enjoy the information, the recipes, and the techniques in this book, and may you have a lifetime of health and happiness ahead of you!

Chapter 1: Choosing Better Health

"A journey of a thousand miles begins with a single step."

- Lao Tzu

Before you can create a weight loss plan, before you can lose an ounce or a pound, before you run out and buy food and supplements and exercise equipment, you need to understand why you want to lose weight. Everyone has a different motivation, but unless you can come to terms with it and make the lifestyle changes necessary for long-term weight management. Losing weight and keeping it off isn't just about seeing a more desirable number on a scale, but about making the mental, physical, and emotional adjustments that will ensure success.

Defining Your Relationship With Your Weight

When you make a decision that your weight is something that needs to be changed, you also need to define why. It's only through this process of self-reflection and self-analysis that you'll find the root(s) of your weight concerns and be able to find a healthy, manageable way to address them. Just as everyone has their own motivation for wanting to lose weight, so too does everyone have their own story about how they gained or acquired unwanted weight.

For many people, age and activity are the number one cause of unwanted weight gain. As we move through life and transition from being active children and teenagers into sedentary lifestyles spent plowing through higher education schoolwork and eventually settle into desk jobs, the time and motivation to go out and work off calories can become reduced. For some, there isn't much time to prepare fresh, healthy food, and the lure of convenience foods becomes too tempting to ignore. Things like fast food, prepackaged meals, and take-out can be loaded with empty calories, sugars, and fats, but being able to have a meal that's ready in minutes can trump the need for 'real' food.

Some people have what would be considered an unhealthy relationship with food. This can include habits like stress eating, struggling with portion control and binge-eating, and not eating regularly to maintain metabolism. These habits can cause weight gain and frequently are based on mental state rather than physical activity. When you stop to think about your eating habits, what do you notice? You can ask yourself:

-When you're stressed out about things going on at home, work, or school, do you reach for a sweet or salty treat for comfort?

- Do you spend all day running around like the proverbial headless chicken, not allowing yourself a few minutes to take in some nutrition, because you're afraid of reprisal or you feel that you 'haven't earned the right to eat' yet?

- Do you have a difficult time leaving food on your plate, because you were trained not to waste anything? Do you instead persist in eating long past feeling full?

- Do you feel the need to continue eating because you're afraid someone will take the rest of the food away, or you feel insecure about when you will be able to eat again?

- Have you ever hidden food, or hidden your consumption of food, because you don't want others to find out how much you've been consuming?

There may be many underlying factors that contributed to your feelings and relationship with food, but if you can identify why you have those feelings, you'll have a solid basis for being able to improve upon these habits. Losing weight is more than just a physical endeavor. It takes work to also overcome the mental and emotional hurdles that can stand in the way of your goals. When you feel overweight, it can lead to self-esteem issues and feelings of inadequacy or lack of self-worth. You don't have to feel that way! You are worthy, and you are wonderful! Weight is a number, and being healthy and happy is more important than being stick-thin. Don't let anyone tell you otherwise.

Medical conditions and the pharmaceuticals needed to treat them can also cause unwanted weight gain. Things as simple as hormonal birth control for women can cause weight fluctuations, and almost any time someone is dealing with steroidal-based treatment plans, some weight gain is expected. Thyroid disorders and other endocrine conditions can also be the culprits behind unhealthy weight gain. Loss of mobility from arthritis and autoimmune disorders can be a physical cause of unwanted weight. New mothers also often find that they've gained weight and lost time to eat properly, leading to health concerns.

If you're dealing with a condition and/or medications that contribute to weight gain, it's important to work with your health care professional(s) to understand why you are gaining weight and how you can alleviate the issue safely. You don't want to create any issues with contraindications of medications and supplements or food. Many doctors will recognize the need to control or reduce weight to improve your medical condition; this is especially true of treatment plans for high blood pressure, heart disease, Type 1 and 2 diabetes, and other conditions affecting the internal organs.

In fact, if you are undertaking ANY major weight loss plan, you should consult with your doctor. Tell them the 'why' of your weight loss goals, and explain what you'll be attempting to do. You might not want to go so far as seeing a dietician or nutritionist, but if you do, your physician can point you in the right direction. They can also recommend physiotherapists or trainers, psychologists, or support groups, and at the very least, give you standards of healthy weight loss that you can use as a guideline to craft your weight loss plan. Your beginning weight, along with your build and bone structure, will give your doctor the tools to help you find an achievable, manageable, safe weight loss goal. While society tries to tell us that thin=healthy, this is simply not medically accurate. Health is tied to so many more factors than your weight, and your doctor will able to help you understand these guidelines.

You should also consult a doctor if you think you may have an eating disorder, such as anorexia nervosa or bulimia. These are real, diagnosed mental health conditions, and there is no shame in asking for or receiving help. These eating disorders can go beyond mental health and affect the internal organs, causing tissue injury and permanent damage, and in extreme cases, death. Please, if you think that you have an unhealthy body image or show symptoms of an eating disorder, reach out to a medical professional. Even if you don't have health care coverage, your health department can connect you with helpful local social services.

Getting Started With Setting Goals

Once you've decided you'd like to lose weight, identified the causes or triggers of your unwanted weight, and spoken to a doctor or health care professional, it's time to set a goal. One of the best pieces of advice that can be offered about setting a weight loss goal is to be safe and be realistic. Keep in mind that the end result is to be successful, so why set yourself up for disappointment?

The average safe goal for weekly weight loss is 1 to 3 pounds. This can sometimes be achieved simply by removing water weight (more on this later), but there's no shame in only losing a half-pound, and there may be danger in losing more through dehydration or food deprivation. The first thing you should do is decide how much you want to lose in total. Ten pounds, twenty, fifty? No matter your goal, write it down. Commit to memory your beginning weight and your goal weight.

The next step in creating manageable stages of your goal is to look at a calendar. Is there a specific event you want to lose weight for, maybe a wedding or graduation ceremony, or the ultimate weight loss show-off, the dreaded high school reunion? If so, you can make that event your goal date. Be realistic and start with enough time to see results, or you may end up feeling frustrated or disappointed in yourself. For general weight loss, stick to the guidelines and come up with a manageable goal date.

You know yourself better than anyone, so once you've set your beginning and end dates, you should then break it down further into smaller chunks of time. Do you want to set weekly and monthly goals? Have a set day for your home weigh-ins? What works best for your motivation and mindset? In the coming chapters, you'll be learning a lot about weight loss methods, and by the end of the book, you'll have all the knowledge you need to craft a plan that includes all the elements necessary for a healthier, lighter, more sustainable lifestyle. Setting your goal weight and goal dates are just the beginning of the journey.

You're going to want a notebook or fitness tracker application or both, and we go into depth later in the book about writing down goals, dates, milestones, mantras, and other things to help you on your way. In the meantime, you can start to think about what type of journal you'd like to keep. For some people, using a pen and paper is the best method, while some are happier with digital means. It's entirely a personal choice, so as long as you decide on a recording method that you will be able to commit to using regularly.

The Complexities of Weight Loss

So far, we've scratched the surface of the whys and hows of identifying the need for weight loss and how to begin creating your weight loss plan. These are very personal considerations, and while they sound simple on paper, they are complex in practice. It can be an easy decision to say, "Hey, I'm not in love with my weight right now. I should do something about it!" but it's not always easy to know the best way to do it, nor can it be easy to get started.

Weight loss has *many* complexities. Understanding your physical health, your mental health, and your emotional health are a great start to crafting a weight loss plan that works. Having the support of a doctor, nutritionist, therapist, and/or fitness trainer would also be wonderful, but you don't need to able to afford these professionals to be able to lose weight. Even if you're not able to seek professional advice at every step, you can be your own advocate and create your own support system. Having someone to rely on for encouragement is incredibly empowering.

Think about the people in your life, and choose one or two family members, close friends, or trusted colleagues to tell about your goals. Talk to them about what you want to do and how you're going to go about achieving your goals. Ask them not to jibe you about having a salad when they're having pizza. Explain your motivations- that you want to feel better, increase self-esteem, have more energy, alleviate a medical condition- whatever it is that you've decided to do FOR YOURSELF, and enlist their aid. When you have a support system, you know that there will be others that can help you through when you feel discouraged. Even if you don't have anyone physically nearby, you can reach out to people on social media or join an online group of other like-minded goal setters. Having support will make a world of difference in your weight loss journey.

Food Is Not the Enemy

Before you start your weight loss plan, it's important to sort out some myths about food, calories, and nutrients. The one problem with food and our human relationship to it is that like any other substance; we can become addicted. Unlike those other substances, a human cannot give up food and expect to survive. Therefore, it's vital that we learn not only about how food and nutrition affect our bodies but to also learn how to form a healthy association with food.

Not all foods, not all calories, and not all diets are created equal. Let's take a moment to examine the word 'diet'; for most, it has a negative connotation. A diet signals deprivation, a struggle to lose weight, and a strict regimen of what you can and cannot have. In actuality, the word 'diet' is defined as 'the food and drink a person or peoples habitually eat,' meaning that diet is and should be tied to lifestyle, rather than a short-term activity. Change your relationship with the word, and you'll change the relationship with the action.

Habits can be difficult to break, and if you identified any bad ones earlier, then you'll realize that the mental challenge of losing weight may be more difficult than the physical obstacles. By redefining the way you think about food, then you'll give yourself a better chance of success. For those who recognized themselves in the question about not 'deserving' to eat yet, have you considered that food is actually the fuel and not the reward? Because it is the fuel, and food is necessary for giving us life and energy. You wouldn't go on a long road trip without putting gasoline in your car, so why are you starting a long workday without fueling up your body?

Calories are a measurement not of weight or volume, but of energy, and your body needs the caloric energy from food to function properly. A calorie is equal to the amount of energy it takes to raise the temperature of 1,000 grams of water by 1 degree Celsius. So what does that science-speak mean for your body? When you eat 100 calories worth of food, that means your body now has 100 calories to use in the form of energy. If you burn those calories through activity, you will maintain or lose weight. If you do not, you may gain weight. It's where we get those calories from that become more of an issue because the body processes different substances at different rates.

Do you remember learning about the Food Pyramid in elementary school? It's an old lesson, but it still has merit, although it's been adjusted a few times over the years as new research comes into play. If you'll recall, it showed you which food groups you should consume the most servings of each day at the bottom, and the groups you should consume less of at the top. These days, the largest group is cereals and whole grains, with a recommended 6 to 11 servings a day. On the next tier is fruits and vegetables, with 2 to 4 servings of each per day, then meat and dairy at no more than 3 servings a day, and at the very top are sweets and fats, which should be consumed in very limited quantities.

This pyramid is a general guide for those who follow an omnivorous diet. For those who say, ascribe to vegetarianism or veganism, the proteins found in dairy and meat products need to be substituted for plant-based foods that have a similar nutritional value. The bottom line is, though, that humans require a certain number of diverse calories delivered in a balanced, nutritious fashion to be able to maintain a healthy weight and lifestyle. While people can be genetically disposed to being heavy or thin, you can have a direct role in your metabolism by regularly following a healthy diet. Let's take a look at the types of diets that are the most common:

- Omnivorous

- An omnivore is someone who consumes everything, as the name implies. Humans are biologically and evolutionarily inclined to eat both meat and plant products, but many people choose to follow other methods for a variety of reasons, including personal, ethical, and religious beliefs, and to address health conditions.

- Vegetarian

- A vegetarian eats a mostly-plant based diet but does not exclude animal byproducts like milk, gelatin, and eggs. A good way to sum up vegetarianism is to say that those that ascribe to the diet don't eat anything made directly from animal flesh.

- Vegan

- A vegan follows a fully plant-based diet, which means no byproducts at all. People who choose a vegan lifestyle often do so for ethical reasons, but many people seeking relief from autoimmune disorders find better health in a vegan diet due to not consuming any antibiotics or hormones that may have been given to the livestock animal. Vegans also try to avoid the use of animal products in all facets of their life, including not using products made from leather or fur.

- Pescatarian

- Pescatarians are those who eat fish and other seafood but do not eat the flesh of land animals. There are indigenous peoples around the world whose cultures are based around their pescatarian diets, and those who ascribe to the diet by choice usually do it as a health-based decision; they are seeking a way to get vitamin-rich protein without the fat content of beef, pork, or poultry. Pescatarians follow an otherwise omnivorous diet.

- Low-carbohydrate

- Many popular diet systems (Atkins, Keto, etc.) are low carb diets, and while some people rave about the results, many say they feel deprived and hungry most of the time. If you are smart about your carbohydrates (more on that later), you don't have to cut them completely out of your life, but this is a decision that only you can make.

- Paleo

- In the past decade, a paleo diet has become popular among people looking to lose weight and get fit, but it's not for everyone. A true paleo diet restricts the consumer to items that were only available before the domestication of agriculture, so this would include fish, wild game, fruit, nuts, and seeds. It's got its benefits, to be sure, because this diet is full of good fats and rich in vitamins and minerals, but it takes a great deal of thought, planning, and commitment to execute.

In the following chapters, you'll be introduced to a number of ways that you can choose to fulfill your nutritional needs, burn more calories than you consume, and learn more about the relationship of the human body to the food it takes in. Having a solid understanding of why these calories are important and how they can be a part of your weight loss plan will help you every step of the way in setting your goals, getting started, and finding a new relationship with food and activity that will be healthy, effective, and sustainable. Let's get started!

"If I really want to improve my situation, I can work on the one thing over which I have control- myself."

- Stephen R. Covey

Chapter 2: Supplements for Adding Nutrition and Curbing Cravings

"Every day do something that will inch you closer to a better tomorrow."

- Doug Firebaugh

When crafting a weight loss plan, some people turn to supplements to aid them in their goals. Supplements are a terrific way to bolster nutrition for picky eaters, help calm food cravings for those who struggle with portion control, and boost metabolism, but they aren't to be taken lightly. There is no one 'magic pill' for healthy weight loss, and it's important to research the effects and potential side effects of any pill or powder you'd like to use.

This is important for a couple of reasons; over-the-counter supplements are not subject to review or regulation by the government, and you want to be sure you are taking something safe. While the government has no oversight, there are both proprietary and independent reviews and studies done on many of the OTC products available on the market today. You also want to make sure that your supplement doesn't counteract or interact poorly with any pharmaceuticals or prescription medications you may be taking.

In this chapter, we're going to be taking a look at the various types of supplements that are available, what their primary functions are, and some pros and cons of each type. Armed with that knowledge, you'll be able to choose if these types of supplements are right for you, and if and when you decide to use them, you'll know how to research their effectiveness and safety.

Vitamins and Minerals

One of the most important things to remember when you want to lose weight is that a balanced diet is best for any lifestyle. Our food gives us more than calories; it gives us the nutrients we need to be healthy, beginning at the cellular level. Humans need a variety of vitamins and minerals to keep our organs healthy and strong. Among many other things, we need calcium to keep our bones from breaking, iron to form blood cells, Vitamin C to boost immunity, and sodium and potassium to maintain our metabolism.

Some people are able to eat a balanced diet that provides all these vitamins and minerals, but the food and supply chain is not the same in every region. There is also, unfortunately, a class discrepancy in food availability, often in large urban centers. Canned foods are exponentially cheaper than fresh foods. If you live in an area that doesn't allow for growing your own vegetables, it can be the difference between having a can of green beans loaded with salt and preservatives and stripped of its nutrients through processing or a fresh green bean packed with Vitamin A and potassium.

Maybe you're just a 'picky' eater. It's a tough label and isn't always accurate. Some people deal with sensory processing disorders where they simply cannot handle eating food of certain colors and textures. Some people have food allergies that disallow them from consuming foods that may be a good source of a certain nutrient. Bananas are a tremendous source of potassium, but if you have an intolerance or allergy for bananas, you'll need to find an alternate source. This is an example of where supplements can aid with both balancing a diet and boosting metabolism.

If you want to start taking vitamin and mineral supplements (or any other type of supplement), there are things you should consider before choosing any products:

- Why do I think I need a vitamin or mineral supplement?

- Do I need to fill a specific need, or do I need a multi-vitamin?

- What are the potential benefits of this supplement?

- What are my expectations of the supplement?

- Has the vitamin I am considering been reviewed and rated?

- What are the potential negative side effects/interactions of this supplement?

- What's the recommended dose/daily allowance of this vitamin?

When choosing a vitamin and/or mineral supplement, it's crucial that you choose brands that have high independent ratings and purity statements. Dosage is also important, and remember that more isn't always better. You don't want to waste products (too much Vitamin C, for example, exits the body in your urine) or swing too far to the other side of health and cause toxicity. Just because a mineral is a naturally occurring substance, doesn't mean it can't hurt you in high quantities. Do your due diligence, and you'll be sure to choose a supplement that's right for your needs and goals.

Herbal Supplements

The use of herbal supplements is as old as human history, but it's only in the last few decades that the science has begun to back up the folklore. There are many ways to ingest herbal supplements, from pills and capsules to powders and teas. Herbal supplements, like many vitamin and mineral supplements, are also not subject to government regulation. This can make choosing these products difficult and lead to confusion. Let's try to demystify some of the popular types of herbal supplements so you can make informed decisions about what's right for you.

Herbal weight loss supplements, in general, work in one of three ways- they help you shed water weight, give your body a serotonin boost creating a sense of satiation, and/or they stimulate your nervous system and quicken your metabolism. The problem with unregulated herbal supplements is learning what doses are helpful or harmful, and knowing exactly how these products will interact with other supplements or prescription medications. Research is crucial to choosing the right product for you. Ask yourself why you want to use an herbal supplement, and then look into what the most recommended herbal substance is for your need.

When researching herbal supplements, the internet can be your best friend and your worst enemy. There is a wealth of information and opinion about these products, and you want to find the correct data. You can go to or call a local health supplements store and talk to the staff there. While their job IS to sell you something, they also are not looking to be liable for selling products that may be harmful. People who work with herbal products every day can be a fountain of information. You should also consult your doctor or pharmacist before taking herbal supplements, just to make sure there aren't any counterindications with your medications.

This advice is not meant to turn you off from the use of herbal supplements, as they can be an effective part of your weight loss regimen. It's simply meant to ensure that you're aware that the lack of regulation means that you should be vigilant about choosing products that have a proven track record, won't interfere with regular pharmaceuticals, and will give you the results you're looking for. Lots of people prefer to use herbal supplements because they are a natural alternative to synthetic dietary products, but just because they are natural doesn't mean you can be nonchalant about their use.

Specialty Supplements

Specialty supplements are in their own category because these are *generally* things that aren't botanically or mineral-based. This could include things like fish oil, supplements for arthritis or joint inflammation, or dietary fiber or probiotics. If the majority of these supplements aren't specifically targeted for weight loss indications, then why are we talking about them? The key answer is because when you are trying to craft a healthy, holistic weight loss plan, you have to look at the big picture.

If you have joint pain that is causing you to be sedentary, then a supplement that addresses and alleviates joint pain might allow you to become more active, thereby increasing your metabolism and triggering weight loss. Similarly, supplements that regulate your digestive system can help you feel more satisfied after meals and be more, ahem, productive in your waste habits. When your digestive system is healthy, it's easier to make food choices that will aid you in your weight loss goals.

When you decide to take specialty supplements, it's so important to think about dosage and side effects, especially counterindications with pharmaceuticals. Many work well in conjunction with prescription medications, but it's always best not to take a risk. There's also the risk of 'too much of a good thing,' especially when it comes to digestive supplements. Intestinal upset is not the healthiest way to lose weight and can cause inflammation and a host of secondary issues. Like with all supplements, it's important to research all angles and talk to any necessary professionals before starting a regimen.

Sports Nutrition Supplements and Snacks

Sports nutrition is big business, and like all big businesses, it encompasses a large market and offers a lot of options. Sports nutrition can be a valuable part of any weight loss plan, even if you aren't an athlete, but with so many choices of powders, bars, pills, and drinks, how can you decide what's the right product for you? Let's take a look at these various forms of sports nutrition and how they work to increase metabolism, replace and replenish lost nutrients, and build muscle.

One of the most popular forms of sports nutrition supplement are powders that you can add to water or other beverages, although some are also able to be sprinkled on food. These powders have varying purposes, but most are protein-based. These protein powders add nutrition and can help build muscle, and are used widely among the body-building and extreme sports community, especially in participants of cross-fit or endurance sports. If you are trying to lose weight and build muscle, you may want to consider one of these supplements. There are also powders that are formulated to help raise metabolism and burn fat.

Sports nutrition snacks often come in the form of protein or energy bars. These are often meant to be used as a meal replacement and offer nutrients in a relatively palatable form that are packed with 'good,' slow-burning calories. They are designed to give you a boost of energy or replace elements lost during intense workouts. While sports nutrition snacks can be a great supplement for people who are leading or attempting to lead a more active lifestyle, they aren't a great long-term meal replacement solution.

Many 'diet' companies also offer lines of snack foods aimed at those who want to lose weight and still be able to have a treat. While these can be nice every once in a while, you should be aware that many contain artificial sweeteners and preservatives. If you're not used to consuming these ingredients, they can cause digestive and intestinal upset. These types of snacks, as well as sports nutrition snacks, can be toxic to pets due to the artificial sweeteners (such as xylitol or sorbitol), so don't share them with your furry friends!

The world's most famous sports drink is, of course, the one with the big "G" and the lightning bolt. It, and others like it, contain sugars and salts (electrolytes) that can restore your balance of hydration. While staying hydrated is one of the healthiest things you can do for yourself *all* the time, there's no evidence that sports drinks are any better than regular water for replenishing hydration. What they *can* do is give you a quick boost of carbohydrate energy to complete your activity and carry you over until you can have a balanced meal.

Like many herbal supplements, sports nutrition pills and capsules tend to function in one or a combination of three capacities: to shed water weight, boost metabolism, or curb appetite. These supplements usually have 'fat-burning' promises in their names or sales pitch. You should be as careful when choosing these supplements as any other. Be aware of the ingredients and dosages, and don't take anything of which you don't fully understand the function and potential side effects. Sports nutrition and so-called 'fat-burning' supplements can have interactions with prescription medications, so be sure to check with your doctor or pharmacist!

Prescription Weight Loss Treatments

If you have done your research and you don't think that over-the-counter products are the right choice for you, then you can speak to your doctor about prescription weight loss drugs. You should be aware that most physicians will not prescribe weight loss pills unless you are highly obese, with a Body Mass Index of 30 or higher, or 27 and above with underlying conditions.

The majority of pharmaceuticals for weight loss focus on curbing appetite or blocking the absorption of fat. These drugs are often not originally created for weight loss; many were tested for other applications, and then it was discovered that they had weight loss as a side effect. Don't be alarmed by this- many drugs are developed the same way, that's why they're called clinical trials. But you need to be informed before beginning any of these drugs, because they tend to have a host of uncomfortable sided effects, including intestinal upset and mental health concerns.

You should talk long and hard with your doctor, your loved ones, and yourself before deciding to take any of these drugs. If you think they are right for your needs and goals, then go for it! Just keep the benefits and potential side effects in mind when you make your decisions, and make sure you trust your doctor's advice.

Now that we've gone over all the basics about the types of supplements available to you, you should have a good understanding of their functions and the questions you should be asking before choosing a product. Adding supplements to your weight loss regimen can be a useful tool, but if you're not sure about pills and powders, or think even with them, you may still need more options, read on! In the next chapter, we'll be discussing meal replacement with smoothies and shakes, how to choose commercial products, and how to make your own at home to meet your tastes, needs, budget, and weight loss goals.

"Motivation is what gets you started. Habit is what keeps you going."

- Jim Rohn

Chapter 3: Mixing it Up With Smoothies and Shakes

"Our greatness lies not so much in being able to remake the world as in being able to remake ourselves."

-Mahatma Gandhi

One of the keys to changing your diet for weight loss is to curb cravings and avoid empty calories. It's not even that we need to eat a smaller quantity of food, it's that we need to be smarter about the food we are consuming. A great way to feel full and satisfied without loading up on fats and sweets is to use meal replacements.

Meal Replacement Options

In the last chapter, we touched upon using protein bars as meal replacements. While these can be great in a pinch, they're an expensive option and aren't always very satisfying past the initial boost of energy they can bring. Shakes and smoothies can be a great way to replace a full meal with balanced nutrition and 'good' calories to keep you satiated while catering to your specific tastes and dietary needs. You can make your own, or purchase powders and concentrates, or even pre-made.

If you're considering making your own, the last two sections of this chapter will address budgeting and planning and give you some basic recipes to get you off on the right foot. It's easier to make decisions about what option is best for you when you understand the function of the ingredients. It's also important to know the difference between a shake and a smoothie, especially for the purpose of learning to make your own. A shake is most often dairy-based, made with ice cream, frozen or refrigerated yogurt, or animal milk (cow or in some instances, goat). A smoothie is most often plant-based, made with fruits, vegetables, and juice, water, or a dairy alternative like soy, almond, or coconut milk.

Considering Commercial Offerings

If you're thinking about the convenience of pre-made or pre-mix options for meal replacement shakes and smoothies, there are some things you should take into account before deciding to add them to your weight loss plan. These items can be costly, and you should be aware that cost and quality do not always equate to results in the realm of weight loss products. Even if you are allocating a portion of your budget that used to go to junk food or fast food, they can still take a chunk out of your wallet if you intend to use them every day.

The best advice I can give you is to do your research. Look for products that are highly-rated by both experts and other consumers. That way, you can feel comfortable choosing something that will give you value for your investment. If you're trying to choose a good powder or pre-mix, be sure to account for needing to buy milk, juice, or a dairy alternative with which to mix the product. Remember, you want an option that will give you true nutrition, not empty calories, so be sure to look at things like sugar content, protein, and vitamins and minerals.

If you're environmentally-conscious, another thing to think about when purchasing pre-mixed or ready-to-use meal replacement options is the packaging. There are many 'systems' available that utilize a reusable container or come in recyclable materials, so those may be of interest to you if you want to avoid excess waste. Many mixes come in large plastic containers that can be cleaned and reused or recycled, and many pre-made shakes come in paper cartons or aluminum cans. Choosing these products can help you save the planet while you work on your health.

One last thing to take into consideration when you're looking at pre-mix or ready-to-eat products is time. If you still need to mix something up, is it really saving you that much time than you would spend making something from ingredients? Is there a way you can carve out time to make a 'scratch' smoothie or shake instead? Making a lifestyle change that is all-encompassing and permanent can mean making adjustments to your relationship with your kitchen, too. Will making a smoothie take more or less time than making a low-quality convenience meal? These are things you should think about when crafting a holistic fitness plan.

Budgeting and Blending for Homemade Meal Replacement

If you've decided that you want to give it a go and make smoothies and/or shakes at home, that's great! But where do you get started? If you've not budgeted for the ingredients before, that's okay, because you're about to get all the info you need to get you on your way to tasty, fulfilling meal replacements made right on your own kitchen counter.

You don't need much equipment to make smoothies and shakes at home, but a good blender will be your best friend. You don't have to spend a lot to get the functions you need, but feel free to go with all the bells and whistles if you can afford to. To be honest, though, you should just look for a model that has a handful of settings, including crush (if you want to use ice instead of water), and puree, because this is the most common setting for blending up large food into a smoothie or shake form. Look around at rummage sales or on your local buy/sell/trade sites; you may be able to find a bargain. Also, consider a scratch-n-dent or floor model from a department store or discount outlet; you might just get a steal on last season's appliances.

Smoothies and shakes should be well-balanced if you're going to use them as a meal replacement. You'll want to make sure they include protein, long-burning carbohydrates and sugars, and a modicum of good fats to aid in nutrient absorption. Fresh produce can be expensive, but there are ways to get more for your money at the supermarket or farm stand. While it's cheaper to buy in bulk, try to avoid purchasing more fresh vegetables than you can realistically use before they go bad. You don't want to 'save' money and then throw it away later.

Frozen options are awesome because you don't need to worry about them going bad before you can you eat them, but try to choose products that say "fresh-frozen" or "flash-frozen" on the package. This means they were harvested and frozen before any significant loss of nutrients. Frozen fruits also tend to be a bit sweeter than fresh fruits, as the sugars are concentrated and released during the freezing and thawing process. You can also purchase fresh fruit and freeze it yourself at home. This works very well for berries, in particular.

You should begin with about a cup of fresh or frozen fruit, either small or chopped small, to promote easier blending. This will provide a natural sweetness without the need to add additional sugars and help keep calories down. Next, you'll want to add your veggies, about a half-cup, again either fresh or frozen. Vegetables add vitamins, minerals, and antioxidants (good for cell renewal) to your mixture. Next, you'll want to add some good fats, about a tablespoon or two. This could be flax seed, nuts or nut butter, avocado- stick with something plant-based. These also add a little bit of protein, which is never a bad thing!

The next part will determine whether your concoction is a smoothie or a shake, and that's your liquid. If you are using milk or yogurt to make a shake, you'll want to add about a half-cup and try to stick to low-fat or non-fat varieties. If you're making a smoothie, you'll also want to use about a half-cup of liquid. Try to use juice without artificial sweeteners, and the same goes for using unsweetened plant-based 'milks.' For shakes, you'll be getting protein from the dairy, but for smoothies, you can toss in a scoop of protein powder to give it a nutrient boost. There's no need to add additional calories when the fruit should be doing the trick to keep your drink from being sour or bland.

Be sure that you've got all your ingredients in the blender and the cap on nice and tight before you push the button! If you like, you can start with your liquid and then add your solid ingredients one at a time until you've got everything broken down and well-mixed. You should avoid running a dry blender, as having liquid in the pitcher lubricates and protects the blades. If you've blended up, and you think your smoothie of shake looks a bit skimpy, trick the eye by adding a handful of ice cubes. The ice will add bulk and hydration without adding calories. The key is to make a filling 'meal' without filler calories. By sticking to the ratio, you can craft a nearly unlimited amount of flavor creations that are sure to taste great, control empty calories, and be a satisfying 'meal' experience. To recap before we get into some recipes, your meal replacement shake or smoothie should include:

- 1 cup fresh or frozen fruit

- ½ cup fresh or frozen vegetables

- 1-2 tbsp. of plant-based fats

- ½ cup of liquid (dairy for shakes, non-dairy for smoothies)

- Add ice for bulk without calories

- Add protein powder to boost nutrients in smoothies

- Try to avoid additional sweeteners, fats, or empty calories by choosing ingredients with no added sugars, fats, or fillers

Smoothies and Shakes for Every Palate

If you're not sure how to get started, here are a few recipes you can use to spark your taste buds and your creativity with your blender! All of these recipes will include a dairy and non-dairy option so you can decide if you'd like them to be shakes or smoothies- once you've tried them, you can start customizing to fit your personal preferences. Remember, it's okay to use fresh or frozen produce in any of these recipes, whatever fits your budget best is perfectly fine. The other thing to remember is, the smaller the pieces, the better the blend, so don't be afraid to take a few minutes to chop up larger fruits and veggies.

Tropical Paradise

This recipe will make you feel like you're on a relaxing island vacation- even in the middle of a crazy work week in winter! Packed with tropical flavor and tons of immune-boosting vitamins, it's sure to make you feel full and put a smile on your face.

Ingredients:

- ½ cup diced pineapple

- ½ cup diced mango or banana

- ½ cup shredded/diced carrots

- 1 tbsp. flax seeds or chopped cashews

- ½ cup plain non-fat yogurt (shake)

    -or-

- ½ cup orange juice or coconut water (smoothie)

- ½ tsp. pure vanilla extract

- handful of ice cubes (optional)

Very Berry Bounty

This recipe feels like an early summer morning, packed full of berries rich in antioxidants and vitamins. This is one you'll return to again and again to satisfy your stomach and your sweet tooth.

Ingredients:

- ½ cup raspberries and/or blackberries

- ½ cup chopped strawberries

- ½ cup chopped baby spinach

- 1 tbsp. almond butter

- ½ cup low-fat milk (shake)

    -or-

- ½ cup unsweetened almond or soy milk (smoothie)

- handful of ice cubes (optional)

Lean Green Protein

This recipe is full of power and protein. Don't let the color fool you- it might look like toxic ooze, but your body will thank you for loading it up with antioxidants, protein, and fiber!

Ingredients:

- ½ cup diced green apple

- ½ cup diced cucumber

- ¼ cup chopped kale

- ¼ cup chopped baby spinach

- 2 tbsp. flax or chia seeds

- ½ cup low-fat milk (shake)

    -or-

- ½ cup soy milk (smoothie)

- handful of ice cubes (optional)

Fruit and Veggie Medley

If you're looking to add a little kick to your routine, this recipe will surprise you! Rich with vitamins and antioxidants, it's sure to a favorite if you can't decide whether you love fruits or veggies more.

Ingredients:

- ½ cup chopped strawberries

- ½ cup diced red apple

- ½ cup shredded or diced carrots

- ½ cup diced beets

- 1 tbsp. flax seeds

- ½ cup low- or non-fat plain yogurt (shake)

    -or-

- ½ cup almond or soy milk (smoothie)

- dash of ground black or red pepper

- handful of ice cubes (optional)

Delightful Day Spa

Everyone loves a trip to the spa- just the smell of the clean, fluffy towels and aromatic oils can bring a sense of relaxation. This recipe will make you feel like you are miles away from home, resting pool-side in a monogrammed robe.

Ingredients:

- ½ cup chopped cantaloupe or honeydew melon

- ½ cup diced cucumber

- ½ cup chopped baby spinach

- 1 tbsp. chia seeds

- ½ cup low- or non-fat vanilla yogurt (shake)

    -or-

- ½ cup unsweetened almond milk or coconut water (smoothie)

- handful of ice cubes (optional)

Colorful Candy Shop

Sweet tooth? This one's for you- with bright flavors and a fun, deep pink color, this one satisfies all the senses without the guilt! We swear it's just as healthy as the green protein recipe.

Ingredients:

- ½ cup diced green apple

- ½ cup chopped strawberries

- ½ cup diced beets

- ½ cup chopped cashews or almonds

- 1 tsp. raw honey

- ½ cup low-fat milk (shake)

    -or-

- ½ cup unsweetened soy or almond milk (smoothie)

- handful of ice cubes (optional)

And there you have it- six recipes to get you on your way to being a shake and smoothie pro! Even if you're not crazy about any of these flavor combinations, these recipes give you a great basis for understanding 'the formula' and creating recipes of your own that you'll love and will keep you coming back for more!

"Food is not the problem. It's what we do with food that becomes the problem."

- Joyce Meyer

Chapter 4: Intermittent Fasting: Not *What* You Eat, But *When* You Eat

"Our goals can only be reached through a vehicle of a plan, in which we must fervently believe, and upon which we must vigorously act. There is no other route to success."

- Pablo Picasso

A popular term that gets thrown around a lot is 'intermittent fasting,' but there can be some confusion as to what exactly it means and how it can be used to further your weight loss goals. To clarify the term, intermittent fasting is a method of eating in which you only eat within a certain time period each day, and are limited to water and unsweetened drinks, like black coffee or tea, outside of those hours.

The key to successful intermittent fasting is to train your body to expect the calories when you take them in, burn them accordingly, and then begin to burn your body's fat stores during your times of fast. This is known as ketosis- but you don't need to be on a ketogenic diet to put your body into this state- it works with any diet plan, be it keto, low-carb, vegetarian, etc. Even without ketosis, fasting can help you learn to discipline your brain and your digestive system to expect food regularly, shrink your stomach, and boost metabolism by leveling out your calorie consumption.

Getting Started With Intermittent Fasting

One of the keys to success with intermittent fasting is patience. Your body will not adjust to it overnight, and you will have to give it time to take hold and begin to work as intended. There are varying time frames of intermittent fasting, from 12/12 (twelve hours to fast, 12 hours to eat) all the way up to 20/4. 20/4 intermittent fasting is not recommended for the 'general population' and is mostly used by those in fitness vocations such as professional bodybuilding. The most popular time frame for intermittent fasting is 16/8.

An example of using 16/8 intermittent fasting would be to wake up at 8 a.m., have a cup of black coffee or tea, and then begin your eating timeframe at 10 a.m. You could then have a balanced breakfast, a light lunch, and a solid dinner, finishing at 6 p.m. The rest of the evening, you could have water or decaffeinated black tea or coffee. The biggest problem that people have getting started with intermittent fasting is the time it takes for their bodies to adjust to the schedule. If you are used to eating at any hour, anything you want, your body won't be happy about suddenly being cut off from 24-hour food intake.

To be honest, and we're all about being honest in this book, you're going to feel hungry at first. But if you truly think that intermittent fasting fits into your weight loss plan, you don't have to start big. If you've been a person who just eats at all hours, using intermittent fasting can be a great way to train your body into eating (and expecting to eat) at regular mealtimes. This means you could go from being a midnight-snacker and late-lunch grabber to a standard breakfast eater! This book is all about lifestyle change, and what a transformation that would be before you even lose an ounce!

Making the Transition

When you decide to make a change and begin intermittent fasting, you should first choose a day to start. You can plan ahead and pick up groceries that are going to be the things you want to eat (much more on meal planning later!) because if you can only eat for a short period every day, you'll want to have the things you like on hand. It can be difficult to change your relationship with your food overnight- we know that feeling! Everyone has had food regret or feared missing out on something delicious.

As you look toward your first day of intermittent fasting, it's up to you to decide what your starting timeframe will be and where you'd like to end up. If you are scared to jump right in, try an 8/16 timeframe. Lay out specific snack times and mealtimes and decide that you will only eat from 8 a.m. to midnight. Don't let yourself eat breakfast early or have just a little late-night snack. You have a whole 16 hours in which to eat, so focus on that instead of focusing on not being able to eat the other eight hours- you should be asleep then, anyway!

You can gradually work towards getting your fasting/eating ratio up to your target by moving the parameters an hour each week. If you started with 8/16, move to 9/15, then 10/14, 11/13, and so on, until you get to that golden ratio of 16/8. Once you begin, it will get easier with each passing week. By gradually working your way toward your intermittent fasting goal, you can help alleviate some of the hunger and food cravings that come with the adjustment to a new food schedule.

Another advantage of intermittent fasting is that it helps you create a more regimented approach to mealtimes and can help you form discipline habits that you can apply to other areas of your life. If you try and 'hoard' all your calories until the end of your eating cycle, not only will you be hungry all day, but you'll tend to eat too much at once, spiking your blood sugar and potentially causing an energy crash early in your evening. This can have a snowball effect of disrupting your sleep cycle. In other words, when it comes to intermittent fasting, don't be a calorie miser.

Once you've settled into your intermittent fasting cycle, you'll begin to notice a difference in your metabolism. You'll be much less prone to snack cravings, and you'll find that your appetite at mealtime finds some equilibrium, too.

Is Fasting Forever?

One big question a lot of people have about intermittent fasting is, "Do you ever stop once you start?" The answer is, you can. You'll not be locked into a pattern of fasting forever if you don't want to be. It doesn't even have to be an everyday thing. Once you've gotten your body adjusted to your fasting pattern, it's okay to take a day off, because your metabolism won't revert. This means you could pick and choose at will- maybe you don't want to miss a late evening birthday dinner for your best friend, or you'd like to have a piece of cake at a wedding, and it's beyond the scope of your allotted calories.

That's okay! Learning to live a healthier lifestyle means making real-world choices that might not always fit in with your ideal diet plan. Many strict intermittent fasters choose to take off one day a week or every two weeks to let their body rest from the stringency of their fasting. Once you've begun a weight loss plan that you're confident in, you'll also become more confident in your ability to make those judgment calls. So, no, fasting can be forever, but it doesn't have to be. You can use it as a tool in your weight loss arsenal for as long as you like, but you have to give it time to work first.

Be patient, teach your body to metabolize on an intermittent fasting regimen, and then you will be free to continue that regimen, choose occasional 'off days, or you may decide that you've learned enough from the discipline of intermittent fasting to make your own food choices here on out. The nice thing about intermittent fasting is that it's free, and you can always return to it in the future if you like.

Alternate Fasting Methods

If you're intrigued by intermittent fasting, but you aren't sure it will fit into your weight loss plan, you should know that there are alternative ways to get the cleansing, stomach-shrinking effects of intermittent fasting without committing to a stringent schedule every day. This could be because your work or school schedule isn't cut out for daily fasting, or maybe you've got a medical condition that requires you to take your prescriptions with food at certain hours.

You can still employ fasts in your weight loss plan, even if daily fasting isn't for you. There are still benefits to be reaped from using fasting in a different way. You can choose to do a 24-hour fast once a week or every two weeks. You could also employ an alternate-day fast, where you eat normally one day, and use the 16/8 method the next. Try doing this with the even and odd days of the month (evens are for eating), to make it easier to keep track of. You can, alternatively, fast two or three days a week. While these methods of fasting will not induce the ketosis of regular intermittent fasting, you will still learn discipline with meal planning, train your body to expect less food, and boost your metabolism.

Sample Meal Plans for Regular Intermittent Fasting

When you're getting into intermittent planning, it's important that you make sure you're getting balanced nutrition even though you'll only be eating for a certain length of time each day. Below, you'll find some sample plans for easy meals and snacks that you can employ for your intermittent fasting days. You can, of course, adjust the times according to your life schedule, by changing your hours to 11 a.m. to 7 p.m., for example.

Sample Plan #1

8 a.m.   - unsweetened black coffee or tea

10 a.m.   - 1 hardboiled, soft-boiled, or poached egg

          - 1 slice whole wheat toast with a pat of butter or honey

	- ½ cup of mixed berries
	- unsweetened black coffee or tea
1 p.m.	-2 cups garden salad with light vinaigrette dressing
	- 1 oz. cheddar cheese
	- 8 oz. lemonade or other fruit juice
4 p.m.	- ½ cup of almonds
	- water or unsweetened black iced coffee
6 p.m.	- 4 oz. lean chicken breast
	- 1 cup steamed green vegetables
	- ½ cup of brown rice
	- 8 oz. sparkling water
Evening	- water, unsweetened decaffeinated tea or coffee

Sample Plan #2

8 a.m.	- unsweetened iced tea
10 a.m.	- 4 strips of lean bacon
	- 1 apple, sliced with 1 tbsp. peanut butter

                        - ½ cup low-fat or non-fat yogurt

1 p.m.   - ½ turkey sandwich on whole grain bread (include lots of veggies!)

                        - ½ cup whole-wheat pretzels

                        - 1 diet soda

4 p.m.   - 1 oatmeal cookie

                        - sparkling water

6 p.m. .   - 1 small lean pork chop

                        - 1 cup of mixed vegetables

                        - 1 baked potato with a pat of butter

                        - unsweetened black iced tea

Evening   - water, unsweetened decaffeinated tea or coffee

Sample Plan #3

8 a.m.   - unsweetened, black iced coffee

10 a.m.   - 2 sausage links or patties

                        - 1 cup whole-grain cereal w/ ½ cup of non-fat milk or non-dairy 'milk'

                        - 4 oz. of no-sugar-added fruit juice

1 p.m. grain wrap	- grilled vegetables on a whole
	- 1 to 2 oz. low-fat Monterrey jack cheese
	- unsweetened iced tea
4 p.m.	- ½ cup of trail mix
	- sparkling water
6 p.m. bun	- 4 oz. hamburger on a whole-grain
	- garden salad with light French dressing
	- 1 diet soda
Evening tea or coffee	- water, unsweetened decaffeinated

In the above plans, you'll see that you've got plenty of room to use your imagination to substitute in foods that you enjoy. These plans are meant to show you how you can arrange your meals to stay full and satisfied all day. One common thing you probably noticed, is that most of the beverages listed, sans fruit juice, are calorie-free. Sodas and bottled teas can be a large source of empty calories, so if you really prefer sweetened beverages, try to stick to using non-caloric or low-calorie sugar substitutes. A word of warning, though- try to keep your usage of those substances to a minimum as well, because they can cause digestive upset or other health issues.

Don't forget that while the concept of intermittent fasting is that 'it's not what, but when,' you don't have free reign to consume a gazillion calories during your eating cycle. It's still important to be mindful of what you're eating and make smart meal choices. Of course, if you've gotten into shakes and smoothies, you can substitute one for a meal in any of these sample plans. In the next chapter, we'll talk more about making choices and how your body responds. You'll see real-world comparisons and learn how you can still enjoy your favorite things without breaking the calorie bank or creating havoc on your internal organs.

"To climb steep hills requires a slow pace at first."

- William Shakespeare

Chapter 5: Protein, Caffeine, and Everything In Between

"Moderation. Small helpings. Sample a little bit of everything. These are the secrets of happiness and good health."

- Julia Child

You get up in the morning, you pour a cup of coffee, throw in some milk and sugar, and go on your merry way. Have you thought about the nutritional content of those things? How about the 'hidden' ingredients? While we're going to nail down how to specifically read labels and choose portions in Chapter 6, this chapter is going to focus on being a critical thinker when it comes to what you're putting in your body.

In that cup of coffee, there was caffeine (a stimulant), fat and protein (in the milk), and simple carbohydrates (in the sugar). All of those elements combined taste like a delicious cup of coffee, but individually, they have a different effect on your metabolism and your nutrition. Thinking critically about your food and beverages is a great skill to have when you're putting together a weight loss plan. From drinking enough water to limiting fats, there is advice to be had at every turn, but when you know the effects of everyday ingredients, you can make solid choices for yourself when it's time to plan and cook meals, or when you're perusing a menu at a restaurant.

Caffeine, the Classic Love/Hate Relationship

It's happened to the best of us. We're dragging from a long day at work, or need a jumpstart in the morning after too little sleep. We stop at a drive-through and grab a giant cup of coffee, and enjoy every drop of that caffeinated bean juice. It works wonders! The fog lifts, we start getting our projects done, and then, bam! The dreaded tummy rumble and trembling hands. Darn you, extra-large cup of joe!

What is it about coffee, tea, and caffeinated soft drinks that make them both wonderful friends and formidable foes? It's the caffeine itself, and with the advent of popular energy drinks and a coffee shop on every corner, it's become even more important to understand the effects this stimulant has on our nervous systems, digestive systems, and overall well-being.

Caffeine is a naturally-occurring alkaloid stimulant, and not only can it be found in coffee beans, some tea leaves, but also in cacao (used to make chocolate) and kola nuts (used for cola flavoring in sodas). It's also found in some other tropical nuts and plants, which can be the source used in some of today's popular energy-boosting drinks. Because it is a stimulant, you can become addicted to it, because, like all stimulant and depressant drugs, it has the capability to affect your brain chemistry.

For most people, caffeine is a staple. It's natural to reach for a cup of coffee or tea in the morning, and coffee and tea, when drunk black, doesn't have any caloric content. However, the stimulant effect can be more than you bargained for when you consume too much, leading to overactive bowels and shaky hands. Too much caffeine can also disallow sleep, sending your rest patterns into an unhealthy spiral. Some people can experience a sensation that their heart is racing, leading to weakness and shallow breathing; these palpitations aren't always the mind playing tricks- they can be real, and they can be dangerous.

Caffeine can be a beast to get away from, and people who do so find that they experience symptoms of withdrawal, including tremors and headaches. If you want to reduce your caffeine consumption, do it gradually. Wean yourself off by having one fewer caffeinated beverage every few days. Find a fun substitute like chicory, which is made from a root and has a similar flavor to coffee, without the caffeine. Find a brand of decaffeinated coffee that you like, and for tea drinkers, considered switching to an herbal blend or naturally decaffeinated green tea.

These words of warning aren't to scare you away from enjoying a cup of coffee in the morning, but can actually be taken to set the theme for this entire chapter- and that theme is vigilance and moderation. When you are cognizant of the ingredients and compounds in your foods, you can make better choices about how much of them to consume. For some people, reducing or eliminating caffeine can alleviate the symptoms of health conditions like heart disease or migraine headaches. The point is, caffeine is so prominent in daily life that the more you know and understand, the smarter choices you can make.

Water, Water Everywhere

Everyone has an opinion on how much water we should drink every day, but few people take the time to explain WHY water is so important. Yes, we all know that we're supposed to 'stay hydrated,' but what does that mean? The truth is that water has so many benefits for your body that it starts way down on the cellular level. Water provides the structure for the walls of our cells, is a primary building block of blood, and is the medium in which waste is filtered out of our bodies in urine. So yes, water is pretty darn important. We need water to perform the basic functions of life.

Experts have determined that the human body can survive for approximately three weeks without food, but cannot live more than 3-4 days without water. When you are trying to lose weight, there are some misconceptions about water and water weight that we should clear up for you. The body retains water as water weight when it's not metabolizing correctly, not because you're drinking too much water. This can happen when you're not getting enough activity and water pools in the extremities, known as edema. This can also happen to pregnant women, whose metabolism can be all over the map as their hormone levels change rapidly. Edema can also be a side effect of certain medications or a symptom of heart and lung dysfunction.

One way to get rid of water weight that isn't caused by an underlying medical condition or a prescription medication is to drink more water. When you regularly keep your cells hydrated, they will function better. You will begin to pass more toxins out in your urine, your stools will be more effective, and you will begin to see less water retention. You'll even notice a difference in your energy levels and your skin tone and elasticity. Drinking a glass of water before meals can help you feel fuller faster and eat less, and water is one of the only substances that is absorbed directly through the stomach walls instead of being shuttled through the entire digestive system.

So, how much water should you be drinking every day, and what if you don't like the taste of plain water? These are the biggest deterrents for not consuming enough liquids every day- the uncertainty and the distaste. The 'amount' question can be answered with some simple math; you should consume between a half-ounce an ounce of water for every pound of weight. So, if you weigh 200 lbs., you should drink between 100 and 200 ounces of water every day, so a gallon (128 oz.) would fall in those parameters. It sounds like a lot, but in reality, it's not that difficult to do. You can fill a gallon every morning and gauge your consumption that way, or you can get a really good 32 oz. water bottle and make sure you refill it 4 times each day.

For people who have an aversion to plain water, there are alternatives. Remember, for every soft drink you consume (coffee, tea, soda, seltzer), water is the first ingredient. The trick is to not let these be the only drinks you consume and to account for their other ingredients, especially sodium content, that may inhibit hydration. There's a reason they put salty snacks out at bars- the more sodium you consume, the thirstier you'll be, so you'll go ahead and order another beer to wash them down- more on alcohol later, though!

You can purchase flavor drops to add to your water or try some natural fruit flavors like a spritz of lemon juice. Another great way to jazz up your water is by making infusions, like cucumber water- simply slice up a fresh cuke, add it to a gallon of water, and chill overnight. It's a refreshing treat on a hot day. You can also try soaking apples and grapes for a fruitier flavor. If you've got a countertop carbonator, you can make your own seltzers that may appeal to your palate more than plain water.

If the taste of your tap water is your biggest deterrent, you may want to invest in a faucet filtration system or a filtered pitcher. These can be more cost-effective over the long-term than constantly purchasing bottled water, and more environmentally-friendly, as well. No matter how you approach your water conundrum, the takeaway here is just to remember to drink enough, every day.

Proteins- More Than Meets the Eye

When you think about proteins, you probably think about a big, juicy steak or a perfectly-scored piece of grilled chicken. Proteins are the building blocks of amino acids and muscle fibers, and they are crucial for human health. But proteins aren't only found in animal meat- there are a ton of delicious options for proteins and some hidden sources you may want to tap to fit into your weight loss plan.

While animal meat is commonly the main source of protein in human diets, animal products also provide protein. This means things like eggs, which are very high in protein, and dairy products like milk, yogurt, and cheeses. While these are a great source of valuable protein, dairy products can be high in fat and sugars, which is why they are usually recommended in moderation. It's great to enjoy a slice of cheese on a sandwich or have a glass of milk with breakfast, but try to use low- or non-fat products as your palate can handle or adjust to. Habitual whole-milk drinkers may find it takes a few weeks to become used to the thinner texture of 2% milk or skim milk.

In the chapter about shakes and smoothies, we talked about adding protein with nuts and seeds. These are a fantastic source of plant-based proteins, so if you're not much a meat-eater or follow a full vegetarian or vegan diet, tree nuts, peanuts, and seeds can be a suitable alternative. However, these aren't very filling, and some contain a lot of fat, not always the good kind. Where can you get bulk and protein without adding a ton of calories? Beans!

Beans are a terrific source of non-animal protein. Soybeans are used by many veggie-alternative companies as the basis for their meat replacement products, and some feature black beans, as well. Soybeans or soybean products like tofu or tempeh are used in a lot of Asian cuisines and can be cooked in a variety of ways. In the American South, Southwest, and across

Latin America, simple, hearty meals are based on red or black beans and rice. This is because the two inexpensive commodities put together have a balance of protein and complex carbohydrates without a lot of fat.

Lentils are a nice choice, too. Lentils work well in soups and stews or can be cooked and blended into dips and spreads, just like its cousin, the chickpea (garbanzo bean). The chickpea is a staple of Mediterranean and Middle Eastern cooking, comprising such popular dishes like hummus and falafel, although falafel can also be made with fava beans or lentils. Leafy greens like spinach and stone fruits like apricots and avocados also provide a good source of plant-based proteins. However you get your protein, keep it lean and eat it in moderation, and have fun trying all the amazing protein options available to you!

Breaking Down Simple and Complex Carbohydrates

Remember when you were a kid, and you just wanted one more piece of candy, and your mom said, "No more sugar!"? That's because she knew that sugar was going to make you race around and crash into a tired, whiny mess. Why does sugar have that effect, and how can you avoid it as an adult?

Sugars and starches are found in many foods that we regularly consume, and their function is to provide us with energy. The difference between eating a piece of candy and crashing an hour later and having a bowl of oatmeal and feeling energetic for hours is the difference between simple sugars and complex starches, collectively known as carbohydrates. Carbohydrates are necessary for a balanced diet, and eating smart carbs can be a useful part of any weight loss plan.

Choosing smart carbohydrates isn't as difficult as it sounds, because there is a direct correlation between how processed something is and how complex the carbohydrate is. Let's look at it this way. A bowl of oatmeal is a smarter choice and a more complex carbohydrate than a piece of candy because the oatmeal goes through fewer processes to get to your table, leaving your body to do the rest of the work breaking it down. This gives you longer lasting energy and gives you the chance to burn off calories processing the food.

By contrast, a standard hard candy is made from not much more than granulated cane sugar, high-fructose corn syrup, and flavoring. Two of those ingredients are simple carbohydrates, or sugars- distilled down so far from their plant source that you would never recognize their origins if the sugar cane and the sugar crystals or the corn and the corn syrup existed in a vacuum. The sugars have already been broken down into their lowest form, leaving no work for your body to do when you consume them. That's what causes the burst of energy, followed by the crash. Your body gets all ramped up to do some work, does it quickly and frantically, and then feels let down when the work is over too soon.

The takeaway to remember when choosing carbohydrates to balance your diet is to think about processing and to leave as much of that as possible to your body. When deciding which bread to buy or which flour to use for baking, remember that whole wheat flour hasn't been processed as much as white flour. The same thing goes for other carbohydrates like rice-brown rice hasn't had the bran and germ removed, whereas white rice has been processed to remove these nutritious parts. Less initial processing equals more work for your body to do and, therefore, longer-lasting energy from your carbohydrate consumption.

Fats: The Good, the Bad, and Knowing the Difference

Oh, no! It's time to talk about fats, and it's tough to talk about one of the worst 'f-words,' isn't it? Fat is something we're taught to avoid, and it can be difficult to know when it's okay to consume them, and how to do so in proper quantities. Fats are also known as lipids, and lipids carry flavor! That's why full-fat cheeses or salad dressings seem to be more flavorful than lower-fat options, or why whole milk seems richer than low-fat milk.

But fats have functions other than carrying the flavors of some of our favorite foods. Fats are the medium in which other nutrients are transported around the body, they are necessary for the absorption of vitamins, and they act as an emulsifier when cooking or baking, holding other ingredients together with their unique molecular structure. Fats also function as a lubricant and anti-stick agent when used in the kitchen.

There are three main types of fats- saturated, monounsaturated, and polyunsaturated, and they all have a role in a balanced diet. Understanding the difference between these fats can help you make better choices when working on your weight loss goals. Saturated fats are the so-called 'bad fats,' and these are generally solid fats, like lard, meat fats, shortening, margarine, coconut oil, butter. These fats can raise your cholesterol levels and lead to other health problems. You should also avoid trans-fats, if possible, which occur in solid fats that are processed through hydrogenation.

Unsaturated fats come in monounsaturated and polyunsaturated form, and these are the 'good fats,' although they should still be eaten sparingly. Unsaturated fats are usually found in liquid forms, like cooking oils, and in the form of fatty acids in nuts and seeds. These fats can actually help lower your cholesterol levels. Fatty acids can also be found in fish like tuna, mackerel, herring, and salmon, and of course, in fish oil supplements.

Knowing the difference in the types of fats, what can you do to still have rich, flavorful food without eating too many saturated fats? There are several ways you can lower the fat content in your diet while still enjoying your favorite foods, and it only takes a few small adjustments. You absolutely *can* create healthier versions of your go-to dishes with less fat and just as much flavor, and you can make choices when eating outside the home to keep the fat content down, as well.

When you're going to make meat, choose lean cuts or trim away some of the fat before cooking. If possible, choose the oven, air fryer, or slow-cooker over the frying pan and deep fryer. If you must fry, choose liquid fats like canola oil over solid fats like shortening. Blot or drain the excess oil off before serving. When baking, understand the role of the fat as a binder and flavor agent, and use liquid fats when at all possible. You can find oil substitutions for lard, shortening, and butter online with just a few simple clicks. If you simply cannot make Great-Grandma's signature spice cake without using shortening, be smart about how you consume the finished product- small portions and small bites, so you can savor the experience, not the portion size.

Going out to eat can be a pitfall when it comes to fatty foods, and only you can decide if it's worth blowing your calorie and fat budget over one meal. Diners are tough, but choosing breakfast options like an omelet and toast can help you avoid the greasy burger and fries without having to 'settle' for a salad. Ethnic restaurants can offer a wide array of good options, and don't be afraid to ask what type of oil they use for their fried foods. (Note: this is good practice if you have any food allergies because some eateries use peanut oil.) If you're not happy with the answer, you can order something that's not fried.

Even movie dates, carnivals, and county fairs can be navigated without falling into the fried food trap. Instead of a funnel cake, get a bag of roasted nuts to share with your companions. Choose a chocolate-covered banana instead of an ice cream cone, or if you just must eat something deep-fried, opt for fried pickles instead of fried Oreos. You can have lots of fun, not feel self-conscious about sitting out on the greasy stuff, and even if you eat a few extra calories, remember that life is about living, too. We're working on creating a new lifestyle, not just a diet, so learning how to make the best choices under every eating circumstance also means learning not feeling guilty about enjoying yourself.

Fiber, Antioxidants, and Other 'Cleansers'

There's something to be said about the satisfaction of cleaning something and making it shine and function properly. There are things that we can include in our diets to achieve clean living, and while we can start by eating a balanced diet of minimally-processed foods, there are other things we can consume that will also help with weight management and 'cleaning out your system.'

Antioxidants are a good place to start, and they are found in many green vegetables and tree fruits. Antioxidants are great for your circulatory system and can help you look and feel younger with their positive effects on cell renewal. Every cell in your body respires, and the waste products they release into your bloodstream are called free radicals. If you don't eat enough antioxidants, which combat and cleanse away free radicals, you are slowing the cell renewal process. When you consume an adequate or even large amount of foods containing antioxidants, you are giving your body what it needs to fight free radicals and accelerate cell renewal.

Fiber is another substance you want to make sure you're getting plenty of. Dietary fiber can help you have regular bowel movements and stabilize your digestive system. You can get fiber in your diet by eating plenty of fruits and vegetables like bananas, oranges, plums, and dark leafy greens. Beans, whole grains, and nuts also have high fiber content. If you have a history of bowel issues (without a major underlying medical condition like IBS/IBD, Crohn's, or diverticulitis), adding fiber to your diet is a great place to start regulating yourself. You may also want to consider probiotics to further straighten out your gut health.

If you are having trouble with your bladder, kidneys, or if you experience gout, you want to add acidic juices to your diet plan. Addressing these issues with tart cherry or cranberry juices can help your kidneys function better, and remove uric acid from your bloodstream, lowering your chances of a gout attack. Better quality of life and less gout pain will allow you to become more active and add more exercise to your weight loss plan.

These are just a few things to consider when you're thinking about your dietary lifestyle. In order to create a holistic weight loss plan, you've got to consider all aspects of your life and make the changes necessary to address those factors in a way that will be achievable and with attainable goals. You'll find that when you start feeling better and seeing results, it begins to snowball- you'll become more active, make even smarter choices, and soon enough, you'll be at or past your goals and feeling amazing about your progress.

Being Smart About Alcohol

Booze- it's always the elephant in the room, isn't it? If you're not an abstainer, you're probably wondering how you can still enjoy a drink or two while you're trying to lose weight. You can, but let's take a look at some smart alcohol choices you can make to stay on track while still having a wee dram on occasion.

Beer is the big question because it's the beverage of choice for many people. Beer can be loaded with calories, but that doesn't mean you have to give it up entirely. Some widely-distributed breweries have begun to come out with low-calorie, low-carb beers in the last decade or so that's pretty tasty. There's also been a rise in spiked seltzers and lemonades that are lower in calories than beer, if you like carbonation in a can, but it doesn't necessarily need to be beer.

Wine is something that should be enjoyed in moderation at any time, but it's when you're trying to lose weight that you need to mind your vino. Some red wines can be very heavy on calories, and even sweeter whites can pack a caloric punch. You can make your wine indulgence stretch a little farther by making a spritzer with seltzer or sparkling water. It's a great way to make one or two glasses last an entire night out or special occasion.

Hard alcohol isn't for everyone, but it tends to be the best choice in terms of the lowest calories per serving. One ounce of hard alcohol has an average of 80-90 calories, and clear alcohols have lower sugar content, like vodka and gin, for instance. If you'd like to have a mixed hard alcohol drink, don't ruin the calorie count with lots of sweet mixers like juices and sugared sodas; instead, opt for diet soda, seltzer, or sparkling water. It goes without saying that you should also alternate your alcoholic beverages with glasses of water.

Keep in mind, alcohol is not only a depressant, but it can also have a negative effect on your hydration, and in large quantities, cause dependency and/or take a toll on your liver and kidney function. If you think you have an alcohol dependency issue, it should be addressed through proper medical and mental health treatment. Please don't ever hesitate to ask for help. This section was not meant to sanction the use of alcohol, but to show you that you can responsibly enjoy it while sticking to a weight loss plan.

Now that we've gone over many of the elements that make up a realistic daily diet, you are armed with a lot of information that can help you make good decisions about what you're eating and drinking every day. You may be wondering why we didn't go in-depth about salt and sodium intake in this chapter because that's also an important dietary consideration. Sodium intake will be addressed in the next chapter, where we'll talk about reading labels and practicing better portion control. Because salt is a crucial ingredient in many prepared foods, we'll be taking a look at recommended daily values and how to use them to make decisions at the grocery store.

In the next chapter, we'll also be taking a look at some ways to use budgeting and meal planning, show you some great starter recipes for healthy meals that ANYONE can cook at home, and teach you how to be a pro at deciphering food labels and avoiding over-processed foods. You'll be amazed at what you'll find hiding on the supermarket shelves, and you'll be amazed at yourself when you discover what an awesome cook you can be, so let's go get started!

"Strength is the capacity to break a chocolate bar into four pieces with your bare hands- and then eat just one of the pieces."

- Judith Viorst

Chapter 6: Reading Labels and Reducing Portions

"We are what we repeatedly do; therefore excellence is not merely an act, but a habit."

- Aristotle

One of the best things you can do for yourself and your weight loss goals is to learn how to read product labels. The nutritional information that you'll find on packaged foods is a wealth of data about the contents of your food, and it can be a real eye-opener when you start looking at ingredients and making comparisons. In this chapter, we're going to put those labels under the proverbial microscope, including what some of the most popular catchphrases really mean and how you can avoid falling into misinformation traps.

Also in this chapter, we'll go even further with nutritional information and talk about how you can use what you've learned to manage portions and to budget both money and calories at the grocery store. We'll also take a look at meal planning, and how to make effective shopping lists you can stick with to avoid temptation. We'll finish up with some simple, flavorful recipes that use common cooking techniques and kitchen implements, so you can see how easy it can be to make your own healthy, filling meals at home, no matter your level of culinary skills. Let's get started!

Breaking the Code- Food Labels, Ingredient Lists, and Hidden Info

Have you ever read a food label? I mean, given it a good perusal and looked at all the fine print? Most people haven't read a food label too closely since they were a kid reading the cereal box, and nowadays, there is a ton of information on there! If you're not sure what you're looking at, it can seem like a foreign language, so let's take some time to go over the things you will find on a food label and what it all means.

- Product name, company, and manufacturer, with contact information

- Every product on the shelves in your grocery store must have basic contact information on it, including the name of the company which produced it. Whereas produce will be marked with the grower and country of origin, packaged products include much more pertinent information, and some may have a dedicated phone number or email address for questions and concerns. In this modern age, some product packaging even includes a website and/or social media links. The great thing about technology and food production is that consumers now have many options available to them to reach out and speak to customer service regarding specific products.

- Product photograph/description

- We eat with our eyes, first, don't we? We like to choose products based on their visual appeal, and most grocery store products will have either a picture or a picture and description of what's in the box, bag, jar, or can. If there's no picture, there may be a clear part of the packaging to allow you to see the contents inside. This allows you to make a decision based on the appearance of the product.

-Ingredients

- The ingredients list on product packaging is mandated to be listed in order of volume, meaning the first ingredient is the one that is found in the greatest quantity, down to the smallest amount, which is the last ingredient. We previously talked about the amount of processing that goes into a food product, and how less processing means your body will do more of the work breaking down that food. The same can be applied to ingredients lists. The fewer ingredients you see, the less processed the food is. That shouldn't be the only factor in your decision to purchase something (the only ingredients in plain potato chips are potatoes, oil, and salt, after all), but it can be an important thing to consider. Also, take a look at the additives and preservatives noted in the ingredients list- if you can't pronounce it, do you want it in your body?

- Serving size and servings per container

- Product packaging will tell you how large a serving size is and how many servings can be found in the container. This is one of the biggest 'shock values' for some people, who are surprised to find out that their favorite foods aren't supposed to be a single serving. In the next segment, we're going to go in-depth about understanding and controlling servings and portions, because this one little line on a product package can have a huge impact on how you approach your weight loss goals.

- Nutritional information

- The nutritional information that you will find on packaged goods will give you a ton of crucial data. First, it will tell you how many calories each serving contains. This is important for a couple of reasons. Knowing how many calories are in a certain product can help you compare with other similar products and make a smart decision. Calories per serving are also important in helping you understand how many calories you may have been consuming before you chose to start your weight loss journey. This can be an eye-opener.

- The nutritional information also contains what is known as percent daily values or recommended daily values. This will be a list of various macro- and micronutrients, vitamins, and minerals and how much is contained in each serving of the product. In the United States, these values are based on USDA and FDA guidelines for a 2,000-calorie diet. If you are on a weight loss plan, you may be consuming fewer calories, but you can still interpret the data for decision-making. You can read the label and understand that if you're eating fewer calories, you'll be getting a higher percentage of your dietary needs from the product, but keep in mind; you'll also be taking in a higher percentage of sodium and sugar. When you look at nutritional values, you can look for foods that have high recommended daily values of vitamins and minerals, and low percentages of sodium, fats, and sugars. Sodium levels are important because it's an element that must be taken in moderation. Sodium is necessary for maintaining electrolyte levels, but because sodium is a desiccant, it causes dehydration when too much is consumed. It can also exacerbate high blood pressure and other underlying health conditions. When purchasing canned goods, try to find varieties that are labeled as having no added sodium. You can add salt to taste at home.

- *Allergy warnings*

- With the rise of food sensitivities, food manufacturers are now mandated to mark the label with major allergens, such as nuts, soy, eggs, dairy, and gluten. You may also see that a product may not contain those items, but it is indicated that they were made in a facility that processes those ingredients. This is so those with severe allergies can avoid food that might be cross-contaminated. While it may seem a little excessive to some people to see milk labeled as containing dairy, it may not be excessive to people who have sensitivities, but who truly may not be aware that milk is a dairy product. The labeling requirements for major allergens are no laughing matter and have probably saved countless lives.

- Serving suggestions/Cooking instructions

- If you look closely at the product picture or read the side of the box, you may see fine print with the words 'serving suggestion' or find some recipes to inspire you on how to use the product. If it's not a ready-to-eat product, there will also be cooking instructions. There's not much of a hidden agenda here, aside from food conglomerates wanting you to also buy their pasta sauce brand when you buy their pasta. The manufacturers want you to see and read how to best enjoy their product so that you will come back and purchase it again. They spend excessive amounts of money each year on recipe and product testing to make sure the directions and the recipes are both tasty and correct.

- Amount of product (weight, volume, or weight by volume)

- This is another mandated label. Food manufacturers are required to tell you how much of their product you are getting in each package. You might have noticed over the years, that a product costs the same or more as it ever did, but there is less of the actual food in the box? And the box is the same size! They just changed the interior packaging to hold less stuff. Prepackaged cookies are a good example of this; these days, you will find a much bigger plastic tray and way fewer cookies. Knowing how much product is in the package will help you out when we get to the section on budgeting. Whether you are trying to buy a single can of soup or a pallet of yogurt, the unit price will be the metric we'll be zeroing in on for learning how to pay less for more.

- Product claims

- This is where things can get really tricky. Product claims on packaging cannot be false, but they certainly can be misleading. When something claims to contain half the sugar of another product, that may mean that the other product has a ridiculous amount of sugar to begin with. The same goes for claims about calories, sodium, fat, or anything else the product may claim to have more or less of. Be wary and use what you now know about nutritional info to make your own decisions about whether or not to purchase a product. Also, use your judgment on taste to make your choices, too. Would you rather have a full serving of something that you're not crazy about the taste of, or a smaller serving of something you like? (Looking at you, light mayonnaise!)

Now that you're a label-reading pro, it's time to take a deep dive into some of the product information that will best serve you as you craft your weight loss plan. Next, we'll take a close look at serving sizes. Once you examine and compare the serving sizes of some popular foods and snacks, I guarantee it will help you change your attitude and your outlook towards both filling up and cleaning your plate.

According to This, I'm a Family of Four? Learning and Sticking to Proper Portion Sizes

One of the hardest things to learn and stick to when you're trying to lose weight and keep it off is portion control When you learn to read labels; you might be shocked to see that the recommended portions of your favorite foods are quite a bit smaller than you expected or hoped for. The good news is, you don't have to stop eating the things you like just because your portions should be smaller. Many dietary lifestyle changes fail because people feel deprived, and we want to make sure that you never feel as if you've had things taken away from you. That's no fun, and it's not a sustainable way to live.

It's frustrating to look at a packaged food product; let's use a box of a prepared meal like macaroni and cheese for example, and realize that one small box is supposed to be three servings. Who hasn't ever eaten a whole box and called it a meal? This is a prime example of quantity not equaling quality. Yes, a box of macaroni and cheese can be filling, but it totals over a thousand calories, and that's when it's prepared with low-fat milk and margarine. If you use butter and whole milk, that calorie count soars even higher.

How can you still enjoy the foods you love-macaroni and cheese, mashed potatoes, pasta, potato chips, etc., and not break the calorie bank? By exercising portion control and eating those things sparingly or as part of a larger, more balanced meal. If you make a box of prepared macaroni and cheese, portion out the recommended serving size and make yourself a big garden salad with a light dressing to be the other part of your meal, or grill and dice a chicken breast to mix into your bowl for bulk and protein.

Now let's take a look at the serving recommendations on a can of vegetables, let's say green beans. There are much fewer ingredients than on the box of macaroni and cheese (three ingredients as opposed to twenty-one), but the can of vegetables also contains three servings. Even if you eat the whole can of beans, that's only around 50 calories consumed. Taking what you now know about how processed a food product is and which calories are better for you to consume, wouldn't you feel a lot better physically and emotionally if you ate a whole can of beans instead of a whole box of macaroni and cheese?

What about products that aren't packaged with individual labels like meat and produce? As a general rule, one piece of fruit or a half-cup is one serving, and a serving of vegetables is also considered to be a half-cup. Many grocery stores will hang small posters in the produce section with nutritional information for you to look over. As far as meat is concerned, most experts agree that a serving of meat is between four and six ounces. This would be a portion of approximately the size of a deck of playing cards, and you should always try to keep it as lean as possible.

Being able to read labels and make beneficial judgment calls about the contents and quantity of your food is a skill that you can put to use during your weight loss journey and beyond.

There are a lot of practical ways you can apply this knowledge to make sure that even if you DON'T know the exact content of a certain food, as when you're dining out, you can still take steps to mitigate your portion size and calorie intake. There are also ways to 'trick' yourself into eating better portion sizes at home. You don't have to always choose the 'healthiest' option as long as you choose the 'moderate' option.

Let's face it- when dining out, you don't always want to be 'the salad guy.' This is especially true when traveling because part of the experience is trying new things and eating local cuisine. If it's unlikely that you'll travel to a particular destination again, you would regret not taking your opportunity to taste new foods. A great way to keep calories down and still expand your palate is by asking servers if you can try a sampler platter, or order a couple of different dishes to share with your traveling companion. Another thing to do when dining out is to ask your server for an extra plate or a takeout box when your entrée is delivered. Immediately split your meal and put half aside for leftovers, and you'll instantly slash the calories in front of you while still being able to enjoy a piping hot meal. Split appetizers and dessert with a friend, or skip them if you're alone.

You can also avoid too many empty calories by limiting your bread, breadsticks, and free chips and salsa intake while waiting for your entrée;

these things are tempting but high in calories, fat, and sodium. Use your bread plate! Take a couple of slices or sticks, and make them last for the whole meal. If you *are* getting a salad, ask for the dressing on the side. Drizzle, eat, and repeat until you're done with the plate- it's likely that you won't use the whole container. Challenge yourself NOT to. Try not to overdress when you're at a self-serve salad bar, either. The sneaky calories are always in the salad dressing!

Because trying new beers and wines is also part of the dining-out experience, be smart about the calories. Try to drink a glass of water with or between your alcoholic beverages. This will help you feel fuller, stay hydrated, and prevent taking in too many calories from the sugars in these drinks. Also remember, you don't have to clean your plate or empty your glass. Yes, you are paying for the food, and you don't want to waste anything, but you're also paying for the experience. Feeling guilty about the calories, and being uncomfortably full may negate the joy you had in finding a great new restaurant. One last tip about calories while traveling or dining out in your hometown- take a walk after your meal! You'll see more sights, jumpstart your digestion, and start to mitigate the extra calories you probably snuck in with that last glass of merlot or bite of signature cheesecake.

When you're preparing foods at home or just want to have a snack, you can be in complete control of your calorie intake and portion size. When you reach for something salty or sweet, think about how much you realistically need to satisfy your craving. Yes, you could have a rice cake, but you could also have a piece of chocolate, but be smart about it. Break a large bar into several pieces, and treat yourself to one or two chunks. Savor your bites, don't scarf. For salty snack cravings, use a bowl! You're guaranteed to eat more if you eat chips straight from the bag. Take one serving, put it in a dish, put the bag away, and eat your snack, happy in the knowledge that you've had your treat AND saved empty calories.

At mealtimes, and yes, this sounds silly, use a smaller plate and a smaller fork. You will trick yourself into thinking you've got more food because it will look like a larger quantity when the plate is full. Using a fork with shorter tines will limit the amount of food you can take in one bite, meaning it will take you longer to eat. This creates a more satisfying meal experience because you will end up taking the same length of time to finish your meal as you would with a bigger plate and bigger bites. One of the most mentally frustrating aspects of adjusting portion sizes is feeling like you haven't eaten enough or for long enough. There can be a sense of, "that was it? I'm done?!?", and this trick can help alleviate that.

Once you've made a habit of reading labels and recognizing portion sizes, it will become second nature. You'll stop having to think critically about every morsel of food that comes your way, and you'll find yourself naturally doing quick calculations to determine if you want to eat something, and if so, how much. In this way, you'll come to realize that you're making a true lifestyle change and that you're not just 'on a diet.' If you find that you've got a particular problem food- one that you just can't seem to control yourself around- cut it off! Sometimes it's easier to say 'no' than to say 'when.' If you can't see a block of cheddar cheese without needing to devour the whole thing, don't buy cheddar cheese! It's a simple solution. You can indulge your cheddar love by getting it in your omelet on a breakfast outing or have it on a burger at your favorite dinner spot.

The main lesson to be learned about portion sizes and portion control is that knowledge and vigilance are powerful tools. You don't have to stop eating the things you love to lose weight and keep it off; all you need to do is adjust how you think about and consume those items. Make high-calorie items a small part of a balanced meal, be smart when dining out, and focus more on quality than quantity when eating a meal or snack at home. These small changes in your thought process will make a big difference in the long term. A final note about portion sizes- don't beat yourself up if you have a bad day or a particularly indulgent meal. No one wants you to feel guilty about eating the alfredo at your sister's wedding. You probably danced the calories off after dinner anyway.

Planning Ahead With Budgeting and Lists

In the last segment, you might have noticed that the foods we compared, the macaroni and cheese and the green beans, were both processed pantry items. Why would we do this, especially after talking earlier about how important it was to eat fresh, healthy food? The point of comparing pantry items was to bring us into our next topic, which is budgeting, meal planning, and making lists to stay on track.

The truth is that fresh food can be very expensive, and the prices will vary by seasonal availability and with market fluctuations. In the United States and many other developed nations, it is cheaper to purchase canned, boxed, and frozen items that can be stretched into several meals or stored in the pantry than it is to purchase fresh meat and vegetables that can be used for a limited time or only one meal. We want to show you that whether you shop the fanciest grocery store or the deep-discount aisle, you can still craft a diet plan on any budget. Even those with the smallest food budgets can create healthy, balanced meals that are filling and appealing.

Being a savvy shopper can save you money, help you be more vigilant about reading food labels, and teach you about the true costs of food and packaging. One of the things we're going to be looking at here is the unit price and cost analysis. This sounds fancy, but it's really just a way to understand whether or not you're getting a good deal for your hard-earned money. Saving money at the grocery store is something that everyone can benefit from, no matter your income bracket.

Let's talk about grocery shopping as a function. You make a list, you go to the store, you grab things off the shelves, you pay, and you go home. Now you've got a kitchen full of food. Great! What are you going to make with that food? Oh...you didn't plan any meals, did you? Time to take a step back and start at square one. The rest of this segment is going to walk you through being an efficient, money-saving, calorie-minding, darn-near-professional grocery shopper, and once you learn this method, you'll be a smarter, happier consumer.

- Plan your meals for the week

    - Some people take meal planning to an extreme, plotting out every meal that they're going to consume for an entire week with no deviations. Frankly, we think that's great if it's your thing, but it's not necessary. For our purposes, we want to teach you more about thinking about diversity in your diet and learning how to be smart about purchasing your food in appropriate quantities. People aren't dogs; we aren't happy with eating the same meal every day for our entire lives, scooped from the biggest bag money can buy. If you're lucky enough to live in a society with large retail food stores, farmer's markets, and wholesale clubs, then you are blessed with a wide variety of food options, even on the smallest budget. Take advantage of the privilege by not becoming 'food bored.'

- To get started learning to meal plan, you should write down all your favorite foods. Think about the things you like to eat for breakfast, lunch, and dinner, and your preferred snacks. Think about recipes you'd like to try at home and what foods you would need to make those meals. Now shuffle all your items around and come up with some full meals. Try to think about a week's worth of meals, and if you've got any plans to eat out during the week. Jot down if you or your kids have any events coming up that where there will either be a meal provided or to which you'll be expected to contribute food. If you take your lunch to work or school, think about common items that can make multiple lunches all week.

- Make your grocery list

- Once you've come up with a list of things you'd like to eat and meals you'd like to prepare, break down the ingredients you'll need to make them. If you want to make pork chops, brown rice, and asparagus for dinner, write those ingredients down separately. If you've got two chicken dishes on your list, then you can write chicken down once, making note that you need two meals worth of it for the week. When you go through each meal and mark down the ingredients, you'll be able to craft an accurate list. Go through your pantry and check on staples like rice and pasta, and if you are running low, add them to your list, as well. Don't forget to check your spice cabinet, too. If you've set your heart on having tacos one evening, you'll be pretty sad if you find out too late that you've not got any chili powder. Also, be sure to check on your produce and dairy, and if you're almost out, add those items to the list, too. Be realistic about quantity. You can always grab another quart of milk, but you'd be upset about wasting money if you have to pour half a gallon of sour milk down the drain because you overbought. You know your own and your family's tastes and habits the best.

- Check the circulars for sales and coupons

- Once you've made a comprehensive shopping list, it's time to look for bargains and adjust. Start with your favorite store (yes, everyone has a favorite grocery store, and the older you get, the more annoyed you will be when they rearrange items.) Check the store's paper and online circulars to see what the sales are for the week. You want to look at both the fresh food options, like meat, seafood, and produce, and the packaged goods options, like prepared meals, canned and frozen vegetables, and pantry staples. If there is a great deal on things you know you use frequently, stock up! Things like salad dressings and breakfast cereals will have a long shelf life in your pantry and can be expensive when not on sale.

- Be a couponer. There's a sort of victorious feeling that comes from getting a really good bargain. Look for clipless coupons on your grocery store's website and on websites that offer manufacturer's coupons. Sometimes, you can get coupons straight from the source. If you've got a product that you love but can be costly, do a quick search for coupons specifically for that product. You'll be pleasantly surprised at what pops up. Also, don't just throw away the coupons that come with your grocery receipt. They might be worthless, but they may also have an option to take a quick survey for a decent coupon or percentage off offer.

- If you've made your list, checked circulars, and clipped coupons, but still don't think you can afford a particular cut of meat or box of cereal this week, don't despair. Look for a less expensive but similar option, or get something else this week as a substitute. Adjust your list at home so that you'll have to make fewer split-second decisions while you're in the grocery store. Being prepared before you leave home can save you time and money at the store.

- Pick a grocery/errand day

- Consistency is key to any weight loss plan, and being consistent about purchasing and consuming food is part of that. Choose a day of the week to be your grocery day, and stick to it, barring extenuating circumstances, of course. When you always get your groceries on the same day, you'll become more aware of the way you and your family got through your everyday products, and you'll be able to predict the items you'll need every week, every month, and every once in a while. You will be also more cognizant of when your store puts out fresh stock and what time of day is best to get your shopping done.

- Being consistent about when you do your food shopping can help you heal your relationship with food. Remember earlier when we talked about some of the food insecurities that can cause us to worry about where our food is coming from, if we'll have enough, and if some person or force will cut off our food supply. It's a small psychological trick, but if you are worried that you need to hoard something and not eat it, or eat it quickly because you're scared it will disappear before you can consume it, the simple act of knowing and reminding yourself that you can get more on Tuesday (or whichever day you choose) can be very reassuring. You can feel safe in the knowledge that you don't have to hoard or binge anything in your kitchen- all these things are renewable commodities.

- Check brands v. generic, read unit prices, consider realistic amounts

- Name-brand vs. store brand is the world's most universal grocery argument, isn't it? In our house, there are a few things that we MUST have the name brand of, and we're fine with the generic versions of everything else. These days, there's a significant push towards improvement in the quality of generic and store-brand products, and many of these come from the same manufacturers and distributors as the name brands, as companies look to streamline production and delivery costs. The price point difference between the name brand and store brand products can be significant and can save you a ton of money over the long-term. Compare the labels, and you'll see that the ingredients are often exactly the same, and have the same or similar nutritional information.

- Let's take a look at those unit prices we talked about earlier and see how using them can help you make decisions in the grocery aisle. In most supermarkets, gone are the days where items have an individual price label. Because the vast majority of products have a bar code on them, and most markets have bar code scanners, you will see prices displayed on or near the products on the shelves. These shelf tags tell you a few important things. One is the price of the product, the second is the day that price is valid through, and the third is the unit price. That tells you how much that product would cost in a set amount, say per pound or gallon. In general, the larger the quantity, the lower the unit price. So if you want to purchase a jar of peanut butter and you're undecided about which size or brand to buy, look at the unit price and choose the best bargain based on that. If you look at a standard 18 oz jar of peanut butter and the retail price is $3.99, that means that the unit price is $3.55 per pound. If you look at the larger 32 oz bulk jar of peanut butter and the unit price is $3.49, making the jar $6.99, it's definitely a better bargain. Peanut butter is shelf-stable, so you can buy the larger jar confident that you've saved a little money and gotten a food item that won't spoil. In addition, you won't need to buy peanut butter again as soon. Unit prices are a useful tool in budgeting and saving at the grocery store.

- It's important to be realistic about how much of something you need to purchase. This is especially true if you have feelings of food insecurity. It can be tempting to buy an item in bulk, just because it's on sale or because you just want to 'be sure you have enough.' Be mindful of falling into this trap on every item. It's nice to have a well-stocked pantry, to be sure, but food waste is money waste. Buy only the fresh items you need to fulfill your weekly meal plan to avoid throwing away food and money every week. Restock your cabinets with dry goods only when they are available at a good unit price.

- Store cards aren't just for little old ladies, so don't be afraid to use one. These can be invaluable in saving money on the items you buy the most, making the coupons you get at checkout more relevant to your preferences, and accumulating points that you can use for future purchases or get free items during the holidays. Some grocery stores will send you personalized traditional or clipless coupons specifically for your most frequently purchased items, so taking the time to get a card and sign up on the store's website can be worth way more than the few minutes it takes to do so.

- Store your food properly

- When you put your groceries away at home, remember that out of sight is out of mind. Put the items you want to remember to eat where you will see them at mealtimes. This means making sure that your fresh produce, dairy, and meat are on prominent display in your refrigerator. If you must, use the shelves for these items and tuck the less important stuff into the drawers. Regularly go through your long-term fridge contents like condiments and pickled items and toss anything that's gone out of date. If you've purchased meat in bulk to take advantage of a sale, be sure it is well-wrapped, dated, and frozen as soon as possible after storage to avoid spoilage.

- Rotating your items is also an important part of proper food storage. This goes for the fridge, freezer, and pantry. When you buy new things, be sure to move the old forward and store the new things behind. This will help you have a good handle on what you have, what you need, and what you're consuming regularly. If you buy a lot of canned vegetables, but aren't eating them as often as you'd like, stop buying them until you've dwindled your supply down a little bit- even if they ARE on sale. In our house, we don't eat many canned or frozen vegetables during the summer because we have a small garden and are surrounded by great farm stands, so fresh is always an option.

- Don't be afraid to visit more than one store

- That last line above was meant to take us straight into our final point about being a savvy food shopper. While it's recommended to have a favorite local supermarket, it's also important that you know how and when to shop around a little bit. If the rival supermarket in town is having a blowout sale on some items you'd like to stock your pantry with, then, by all means, head over there and take advantage of the sale. Use wholesale club memberships to buy things like bulk beverages and deli meats if you will use them in a timely fashion and have someplace to store them. And lastly, try to go to your local farm stands and farmer's markets in season. You will find great deals on fresh produce and dairy, and you'll feel secure in knowing you know exactly where that food came from while supporting small businesses.

- Form a personal relationship with your food

- Building on the theme of shopping for fresh items at local businesses, there are other great ways to save money and build a real connection with the food you consume. Check around your area for farm shares and/or CSAs (consumer-supported agriculture). You can pay a seasonal subscription price for a weekly or bi-weekly share in a farm's fresh produce. The fun thing about having a farm share is that you get to be creative with the ingredients that come in your box each week. You can usually choose which foods you DON'T want to receive (any other broccoli haters out there?), but beyond that, you will receive what is ripe on any given week.

- Buy a meat share or whole animal from a local farmer. Livestock farmers will offer deals in the spring on young animals that will be slaughtered in the fall. You can buy in part or all of the animal, and when it is processed, you will receive your share of the meat, which you can freeze for use the rest of the year. This usually applies to both beef cattle and pigs, so shop around and find a good price on the meat package you want and never worry about supermarket meat again. Similarly, you can go to a specialty butcher shop and ask if they have bundles you can purchase for a subscription price. In places where deer hunting is legal and popular, many hunters will also sell their venison for the price of covering the butcher or processor's fee.

- Grow a small garden, if you can. You don't have to have a lot of space or time to plant some containers of vegetables and herbs to prepare your favorite foods. Nurturing a plant from seed or seedling through harvest makes you appreciative of the effort that farmers go through to produce your food, and makes you more likely to eat it because you don't want to waste your efforts. Try growing the vegetables you love the most, and some you'd like to try but have a hard time finding in stores. It's a fulfilling hobby with the best reward at the end- fresh food!

- What about subscription meal plans?

- There are a few types of subscription meal plans on the market, and it's important to know the difference before deciding if you have the desire or the budget to purchase them. First, there are daily meals produced by weight loss brands, where you pay per month for all of your food to be shipped to you (usually frozen and boxed), and then you simply eat it on their schedule and supplement it with fresh foods and vegetables. This is great if you are terrible at meal planning and cooking, but it comes at a heavy premium and may not fit your budget. You can buy many of these same meals in the grocery store freezer section for a fraction of the cost. Still, eating these meals doesn't teach you any planning or preparation skills, so if you do buy them at retail stores, don't make a habit of having them for every meal. They can make a good portioned-controlled lunch to have at work, but that's about it.

- Some meal delivery services provide you with one meal per box, customizable to the size of your family, and some set preferences. These can be expensive, but they have their uses if you can afford to get them even once or twice a month. You will be exposed to new recipes and cooking techniques, and this can be a great way to expand your palate and expertise. However, do some comparison shopping before signing up. Some of the boxes are complete meals, with no need to add additional ingredients from home. Some of them are incomplete, meaning you are paying for the box and still need to pay for fresh ingredients like eggs, dairy, and produce. Read the fine print before you buy to determine what's best for you.

- If you don't have access to farm stands or have a way to grow your own vegetables, you can sign up for a produce subscription from an 'ugly fruit' company. These cooperatives collect fruits and vegetables from farms and market gardeners that are deemed too 'ugly' to go to the supermarkets. Like a farm share or CSA, these subscriptions only offer a limited 'do not want' option, so you get what you get and have to be creative about the contents of your delivery.

Phew, that was a lot of information about planning a simple weekly trip to the grocery store and being a savvy shopper! Rest assured, once you make a habit of meal planning, making lists, getting your bargains, and storing your food properly, it will become second nature, and you'll wonder how you ever ran into the store all willy-nilly and just grabbed things! In the last section of this chapter, we'll go through some simple recipes that you can make at home with readily-available ingredients. Have fun with these recipes! Part of learning how to be smarter with your food consumption is taking responsibility for what you're eating, but that doesn't mean that food needs to be boring!

Get Cookin': Flavorful Recipes for Everyday Life

There are a few things that everyone should know how to cook, and then there are those that want to learn how to make things they can adapt to their tastes while learning new cooking methods. If you can boil pasta, make a grilled cheese sandwich, and use a knife well enough to slice your veggies without slicing off your fingers, you've got enough basic skills to learn any of the following recipes. Even if these recipes aren't for you, there are still some things you should remember about cooking for good health-

- if you use fats, use healthy fats, and avoid deep-frying if possible

- don't overboil fresh veggies; steam or blanch them to retain nutrients instead

- when roasting, use a drip rack/pan or larger pan than necessary to pool drippings away from your food, drain or blot any greasy food before eating

- add extra veggies in unexpected places, like pureeing carrots or squash to add to tomato sauce for pasta

- use seasonings rather than plain salt to add flavor without adding sodium

- buy an inexpensive food scale to help you divide out portions that are listed by weight and not volume, e.g., 100 grams as opposed to ½ cup.

With all that in mind, let's get cooking!

Night-Before Breakfast Bake

Everyone likes to save time, and this flavorful breakfast casserole can be assembled the night before and tossed in the oven while you're getting ready in the morning. It also makes great leftovers to have for breakfast all week. This recipe is for a 9" x 13" casserole dish, but it can be scaled down to an 8" round or square pan by cutting the recipe in half, or easily doubled if you want to make more for a holiday brunch or potluck event. This recipe is versatile, so try mixing it up with different combinations of meat, cheese, and vegetables to enjoy new flavors every time you make it. It's also a fabulous way to use up leftover meat and vegetables from other meals.

You will need:

- Non-stick cooking spray

- 4-6 slices whole wheat, oat, or rye bread

- 8 eggs

- 2 cups diced vegetables of choice (try broccoli, peppers, onions, potatoes, carrots, etc.)

- 1 cup cooked, diced meat (try ham, sausage, bacon, turkey bacon, etc., or meat substitutes)

- 1 cup shredded low-fat cheese (try sharp cheddar, mozzarella, Colby, etc.)

- Salt, pepper, paprika to taste

To prepare:

1. Spray a 9" x 13" casserole dish with cooking spray and line the bottom of the dish with bread slices

2. In a large bowl, crack and lightly beat the eggs

3. Add in the vegetables, meat, and cheese, and mix well

4. Mix in seasonings

5. Pour the egg mixture over the bread in the casserole dish

6. Cover and refrigerate overnight

To bake:

1. Preheat the oven to 350*

2. Bake, uncovered, for 20-30 minutes, until eggs are set to your preference and top is lightly browned

3. Remove from oven and let sit for 5 minutes before slicing and serving

*This recipe makes 8 servings. Each serving is +/-350-400 calories based on your ingredient choices

Spicy Morning Burritos

Everyone loves burritos! From the soft texture of warm tortillas to the portability of breakfast on the go, you and your family are sure to love the spicy, savory taste of these morning treats. Play around with the ingredients to find a flavor combination that's just right for you. You can make these burritos ahead of time and freeze them to have a handy heat-and-eat breakfast whenever you'd like. This recipe makes 4 large or 8 small burritos.

You will need:

- 4 large or 8 small whole-grain tortillas

- 1 T. olive or canola oil

- 1 ½ cups crumbled chorizo sausage

- 4 eggs, lightly beaten

- ½ cup diced bell or jalapeno pepper (depends on your taste in spice)

- 1 medium tomato, diced

- ½ cup shredded low-fat cheese (try pepper jack for an extra kick!)

- 1 tsp. garlic powder

- Salt and pepper to taste

- Hot sauce, if desired

To prepare:

1. Heat a large skillet and add oil

2. Sauté sausage and peppers until heated through and lightly browned

3. Add eggs and garlic powder and cook on medium-low, stirring frequently until eggs are scrambled

4. Fold in tomato and cheese, and cook on low until tomatoes are warm and cheese is melted

5. Spoon mixture onto warm or room temperature tortillas, roll up, and enjoy! Try a dash of hot sauce to kick them up further.

6. For freezing and reheating: When burritos are cool, wrap well in freezer paper and stack in a freezer bag; reheat wrapped in foil in a 325* oven for 30-40 minutes or leave in freezer paper and microwave for 1 ½ -2 minutes.

*These burritos are hearty and filling, weighing in at +/-750 calories for the large size. While this might seem like a lot, they can easily be cut and shared between two people (or have half for breakfast and reheat the other half for lunch at work), or make the smaller version and freeze the rest for other days. To cut calories, try using only the egg whites or skip the cheese.

<u>Rainbow Salad</u>

On a hot day, there is nothing better than a big salad for lunch! This recipe makes a colorful, tasty meal with lots of flavors and textures, dressed with a simple bright vinaigrette. With no lettuce to wilt, you can make this salad and refrigerate it to enjoy for lunch all week, or make a double batch for your next picnic to share with all your friends and family.

You will need:

for the salad:

- 1 large tomato, diced

- 2 large carrots, diced

- 1 can of sweet corn, drained

- 1 large or 2 small cucumbers, diced

- 1 can sliced beets, drained

- 1 can chickpeas drained

for the dressing:

- ½ cup light olive oil

- ¼ cup red wine -or- balsamic vinegar

- 1 tsp. onion powder

- 1 tsp. garlic powder

- ½ tsp. ground black pepper

- 1 tsp. honey

To prepare:

1. Dice and drain all your vegetable ingredients and mix well in a large bowl- you want them to be as 'dry' as possible, so the dressing adheres

2. Put all of your dressing ingredients in a closed container (mason jars or clean, empty bottles work well) and shake- shake, shake, shake- until well combined.

3. Pour the dressing over the mixed veggies and stir well to coat

4. Refrigerate at least two hours, but sitting overnight will let the flavors begin to meld

* Each one-cup serving of this salad is +/-150 calories and contains healthy fats, vitamins, minerals, and antioxidants. For bonus antioxidants, don't peel your cucumber!

No Press? No Problem! Paninis

Even when you're on a weight loss plan, nothing hits the spot like a good sandwich. Paninis are a popular choice when dining out, but even if you love them, you may not be too interested in spending the money on a panini press. That's okay because you don't need one! If you've got a skillet (bonus points for having a ribbed one to make the 'press marks') and another pot or tea kettle, you can make perfectly-pressed sandwiches right at home. For this recipe, we're going to make a ham and cheese panini, but you can substitute in any ingredients you'd like- this is all about learning the methodology.

You will need:

for the sandwiches

- Whole grain bread

- Light -or- olive oil mayonnaise (for cooking)

- Sandwich fillings

    - sliced ham

    - thinly sliced cheddar cheese

    - veggies like tomatoes, onions, peppers, pickles- choose what you like

- yellow or spicy brown mustard

*for the cooking method

- one medium skillet (ribbed if possible)

- aluminum foil

- tea kettle or medium saucepan

- tap water

- sturdy spatula

To prepare:

1. Lay out your bread and spread a thin layer of mayonnaise on the slices

2. Heat up your skillet on medium-high heat

3. Wrap the bottom of your tea kettle or saucepan in aluminum foil, just to keep it and your sandwich clean

4. Place a slice of bread, mayo side down, in the hot skillet and quickly build your sandwich

5. Cover the sandwich with a second slice of bread, mayo side out

6. Fill your kettle or pan with water and set it on top of your sandwich- the weight of the water acts as the 'press'

7. Grill three minutes, remove the kettle/pan and flip the sandwich

8. Place the 'press' back on and grill for four minutes

9. Repeat 2 minutes each side if you like your bread darker

10. Slice, serve, and enjoy!

* The average homemade panini sandwich is +/- 400 calories, but this will vary based on your choice of ingredients. Use low-fat cheeses and keep condiments to their recommended servings to avoid blowing up the calorie count.

Got Beans? Soup

Making and eating soup is such a comforting activity, and it's even better when it's healthy, full of antioxidants and fiber, and relatively guilt-free. This is a great recipe for a bean soup that's easy to adapt to your tastes, and it also freezes well for meal planning. The ingredients below will use navy beans, but you can substitute any dried beans that you like or have floating around in the pantry. This recipe is vegetarian, but feel free to serve with a sprinkle of crumbled bacon or diced ham.

You will need:

- 1 32 oz. container of no-sodium vegetable broth

- 8 cups water

- 1 28 oz. can tomato puree

- 2 bags dried navy beans

- 2 cups diced carrots

- 2 cups diced potatoes

- 2 T. Italian seasoning mix

- 2 T. dried minced onion (optional)

- Salt and pepper to taste

To prepare:

1. To make the stock, combine vegetable broth, water, tomato puree, and Italian seasoning in a large stockpot; this includes the minced onions if you are using them

2. Bring the stock to a boil and add beans, boil hard for ten minutes

3. Reduce heat to medium-low and simmer for one hour, stirring occasionally

4. Add carrots and potatoes, and continue to simmer and stir until all the vegetables are tender, about one hour; add salt and pepper to taste during this step

5. Serve hot with a sprinkle of fresh, dried oregano or parsley for garnish

6. To freeze, let the soup cool completely and portion out into airtight bags, jars, or containers, and make sure to put the date on the containers before freezing

* A two-cup bowl of bean soup contains +/- 325 calories and is a filling way to get antioxidants and fiber.

Easy Cheesy Meatloaf

Another comfort food that you can adapt to your tastes and nutritional needs! By using ground turkey, this meatloaf delivers all of the flavor and texture of a traditional beef meatloaf while saving calories and fat. Baking the loaf in a round pan instead of a loaf pan also allows the fat drippings to run off, making it both easier to serve and less greasy! It's a win-win.

You will need:

- 2 lbs. lean ground turkey

- ½ c. seasoned breadcrumbs

- ½ c. pasta or tomato sauce

- 2 large eggs

- ½ cup shredded low-fat mozzarella or Italian-blend cheese

- 1 tsp. garlic powder

- 1 tsp. onion powder

- Salt

- Italian seasoning or vegetable seasoning spice blend

- Non-stick cooking spray

To prepare:

1. Preheat the oven to 375* and spray a medium-size cast-iron skillet or round baking pan

2. In a large bowl combine the meat, breadcrumbs, sauce, eggs, cheese, garlic, and onion

3. Mix with CLEAN hands until fully incorporated

4. Form mixture into a high oval loaf in your prepared pan, leaving room around the edge for drippings

5. Sprinkle salt and seasoning blend to taste on top of the loaf

6. Bake, uncovered for 1 hour (60 minutes)

7. Let rest for 5 minutes before slicing

*This meatloaf makes 6-8 slices, which will be +/- 200-250 calories apiece. It can also be sliced, frozen, and reheated to make meal planning easy, or prepared and frozen for up to a week in advance of cooking. Allow a full frozen meatloaf to thaw completely before baking according to original instructions.

Veggie Tots

Who doesn't love tater tots? Those golden nuggets of crispy potato are delicious and so much fun to eat. But what if you could make tots out of other things right in your own kitchen, and what if those tots could be prepared and frozen ahead of time so you could enjoy them on your own schedule? Veggie perfection.

You will need:

- 4 cups finely shredded vegetables (try squash, zucchini, carrots, or any mixture you like!), rinsed and well-drained

- 1 cup seasoned breadcrumbs

- 2 T. olive oil

- 2 tsps. garlic powder

- 1 tsp. salt

- 1 tsp. ground black pepper

To prepare:

1. Pat vegetables with a paper towel to remove as much excess moisture as you can

2. Mix all ingredients in a large bowl; use your CLEAN hands if necessary

3. Line a baking sheet with parchment, freezer, or wax paper

4. Using a teaspoon or melon-baller, scoop out small balls of vegetable mixture and place on the baking sheet

5. Freeze the sheet for minimum 2 hours, overnight if possible

6. Peel the tots off the sheet and store in a labeled freezer bag

To heat and enjoy:

1. Preheat the oven to 425*

2. Place frozen tots in a single layer on a baking sheet

3. Cook for 10-15 minutes, then give the sheet a shake or turn the tots

4. Cook for 5-10 more minutes until the tots are lightly browned

5. Serve with your favorite condiment for dipping (BBQ sauce and honey mustard work well)

*Each tot is +/- 20 calories for the purpose of planning your servings. While standard tater tots have a similar calorie count, they are much higher in fat and carbohydrates than those made from non-starchy vegetables.

No-Guilt, No-Bake Greek Yogurt Mini Cheesecakes

Dessert is the best part of the meal, but it's hard to think about dessert without thinking about all the empty calories it can bring. Cheesecake evokes a sense of decadence, but with these little treats, you can experience that richness with far fewer calories than a traditional cheesecake recipe.

You will need:

- 12 vanilla wafer cookies

- 8 oz. low-fat cream cheese

- ¾ cup non-fat Greek yogurt

- ½ cup honey

- 3 T. lemon juice

- 1 tsp. vanilla extract

- berries for garnish

To prepare:

1. Line a 12-count muffin pan with cupcake papers, and place a vanilla wafer cookie in each spot

2. In a large bowl, combine cream cheese, yogurt, honey, lemon juice, and vanilla

3. Using a hand mixer or stand mixer, beat on medium-high until mixture is smooth and creamy

4. Spoon filling into cupcake liners, then gently shimmy the pan to level the cups and release any air bubbles

5. Refrigerate overnight, and serve with a spoonful of fresh or frozen berries

6. Mini-cheesecakes can be stored in an airtight container in the fridge for up to a week

*While there are few desserts that are low calorie, this one does pretty well for itself at +/- 130 calories per serving. These are rich enough to be filling and small enough to not break the calorie bank.

Sherbet Parfait

Frozen desserts can hit the spot any time, but especially on a hot summer day. Ice cream can be tasty, but it's full of fats and empty calories. What if you could make rainbow sherbet, at home, without too much processed sugar, and without an ice cream maker? It's like a grown-up version of that nostalgic classic and is sure to please whether you make it for yourself to last for a while, or to share at a party.

You will need:

- 3 cups of low- or non-fat milk, or non-dairy milk substitute

- ½ cup granulated sugar

- ½ cup of honey

- 1 packet each of 3 unsweetened soft drink powder flavors (try raspberry, orange, and grape, etc.)

- 3 cups frozen mixed berries

- fresh mint for garnish

To prepare:

1. In a large mixing bowl, combine milk, sugar, and honey

2. Beat on high for three minutes until frothy

3. Split the mixture into three shallow dishes

4. Add 2 tsps. of soft drink powder to the dishes (1 flavor per bowl)

5. Place the dishes in the freezer and let set for two hours

6. Remove the bowls from the freezer; place Flavor #1 in the mixing bowl and beat on high for two minutes to become creamy

7. Place Flavor #1 back in its dish in the freezer, repeat for Flavors #2 and #3

8. Freeze all flavors overnight

To plate and serve:

1. Remove your sherbet from the freezer and let soften for a few minutes

2. Scoop Flavor #1 into a clear glass dish, like a parfait bowl or trifle dish

3. Top with a layer of frozen fruit

4. Repeat with Flavors #2 and #3

5. Set back in the freezer until it's time to serve, garnish in a dessert bowl with a sprig of fresh mint

* A one-cup serving of this dessert is +/-175 calories, but it's likely that you won't eat it a full cup at a time. This treat is fun, classy, and easily adjusted to any flavor or color to have superb visual appeal at parties!

We hope you have a ton of fun preparing and adapting these recipes to your personal tastes! Cooking can be relaxing and rewarding when you know that the end result will be delicious and nutritious. In the next chapter, we'll be looking at other ways to relax and get connected with some inner peace to help you keep stress levels down and stick to your weight loss plan.

"If you can't fly then run, if you can't run then walk, if you can't walk then crawl, but whatever you do you have to keep moving forward."

- Martin Luther King, Jr.

Chapter 7: Calm Down! Reducing Stress to Lose Weight

"Happiness is a butterfly, which when pursued, is always beyond your grasp, but which, if you will sit down quietly, may alight upon you."

- Nathaniel Hawthorne

S-T-R-E-S-S!!! We are all stressed out. Pressures at work and school, tensions at home and in personal relationships, and our own insecurities and anxieties can have us feeling drained, overwhelmed, and out of control. You may not feel like this all the time, but when you do, it can be a whammy on your eating and sleeping schedules, which in turn, can · set your metabolism into a tailspin. In this chapter, we're going to address the different ways that mental and emotional stress can manifest itself physically, and what you can do to keep yourself on track with your weight loss strategy even while outside stimuli try to derail you.

You Can't Metabolize Properly When You're Panicking!

When we're stressed out, our bodies can feel under assault and shut down our metabolisms as a defense mechanism. This is a normal, evolutionary response to being under attack, but it can wreak havoc on a weight loss plan. The human body tends to skew to extremes when under mental and emotional distress, and that is to completely erase the appetite or to start pumping out stress hormones like cortisol that prevent weight loss by retaining fat 'just in case' the threat doesn't go away. Don't be mad; your body is doing what it was designed to do. You just need to find a way to handle the stress and get yourself back on track.

These can be frustrating circumstances. Not only are you feeling overwhelmed by whatever stimuli are causing your distress, but now you're feeling like your weight loss plant is also being negatively affected. Of course, it's tough to calm down when it feels like everything is going awry, so don't focus on calming down overall. Pick one thing you can control or find a solution for, and fix it. When you begin to feel more in control, your mental state and your metabolism will begin to become more normalized. Keep working on your life, one little thing at a time, while doing your best to stick to your plan. Even if you don't feel like eating, try to eat something small and nutritious. You don't want your metabolism to shut down because it's worrying that it won't get fed again soon. It's just as damaging for your metabolism to not eat as it is to overeat.

Please Don't Eat Your Feelings

The flip side of skipping meals when you're stressed out is emotional eating and overeating. We are all guilty of this from time to time- a really bad day at work, and somehow bag of potato chips will make it all go away. Comfort food is a real psychological phenomenon, and while an occasional indulgence shouldn't set back your entire weight loss plan, you don't want to make a habit of it.

We emotionally eat to fill a void, both physical and mental; sorry to be so blunt! When we eat comfort food, it triggers memories of feeling warm, safe, or happy. You can retrain yourself to reach for healthier snacks to get that same feeling of warmth or find something other than food to assuage your feelings. The idea is to be able to know the difference between true hunger and emotional hunger. True hunger develops over the normal course of time, but emotional hunger can strike in sudden cravings, which can have you feeling frantic if you don't indulge them. This is caused by fluctuating hormones, which is also a cause of cravings in pregnant women.

When you feel like you absolutely MUST reach for a bag of chips, take a short walk to clear your head and boost your metabolism. Find a new hobby, one that calms you down and makes you step away from your stressors and your refrigerator. Try knitting! It's inexpensive and productive, and even if you only learn a couple of basic stitches, you can bang out scarves and blankets for your entire family! Hobbies that require focus and repetitive motion can be very soothing when you need to reset your emotions.

Stress, Insomnia, and Losing Weight; An Uphill Internal Battle

It can be difficult to sleep when we're under a lot of stress. Heck, it can be difficult to sleep even when we're feeling like life is going okay. One of the hardest things to remember, especially as adults, it that sleep is a crucial part of being healthy and letting our bodies rest and repair themselves. Unfortunately, in the fast-paced world we live in, it's almost a competition to see who can function on the smallest amount of sleep. This simply isn't a healthy approach, and we need to move past the notion that lack of sleep is a badge of honor to be earned.

When we don't get enough sleep, there are mental, emotional, and physical implications. We don't think clearly, we feel edgy and defensive, and our systems just can't seem to regulate themselves. If you are on a weight loss plan, sleep becomes even more important to stabilizing metabolism, renewing cells, and regaining stamina. It can be so easy to fall into a cycle of not sleeping well enough, and stress does nothing to improve that cycle, so let's take a look at some ways you can find some calm, create a bedtime routine, and get the rest your body desperately needs to repair and renew itself to optimize metabolism.

First, lay off the caffeine late in the day. If you're a coffee drinker at work, leave it at work. Try not to consume any caffeinated beverages after dinner, and certainly not as the evening wears on. Caffeine can overstimulate you and make you feel jittery, increasing late-night anxieties, and insomnia. Instead, try an herbal tea blend with lavender and/chamomile to help you relax and unwind.

Try to turn off screens an hour before bedtime, to let your eyes rest, and help your system recover from being bombarded by blue light all day. It hits us from our computer, tablet, phone, and TV screens, and alerts our bodies that there is something we need to pay attention to, and takes a while to unwind from. If you are a person that needs stimulation until your eyes are too heavy to stay open, read a traditional paper book or magazine, doodle in an adult coloring book, or crack open a crossword puzzle booklet. If you need noise to fall asleep, try a white noise machine or listening to music rather than watching TV.

The temperature of your bedroom also plays a big role in getting proper sleep. If it's too warm, your body will expend energy trying to cool itself down, and even if you can get to sleep, you'll toss and turn, and it won't be the sort of restful sleep your metabolism needs to recover. Try sleeping in a cooler room, cold if possible. It's much easier to toss on an extra cover to feel comfortable than it is to try to cool off. You can also try taking a warm shower before bed to regulate your body temperature, help you feel relaxed, and keep you away from screens for a while before you lay down.

Aging, Hormones, Stress, and Weight Loss

Remember a time when 'middle-age spread' was a common term? The truth is, middle-age weight gain is more attributed to stress than it is to age, but it's still a very real thing. As we mature, our bodies naturally fill out, our metabolism slows down, and our hormones fluctuate. But much of our hormone fluctuation is caused by outside stress hastening our natural biological processes. Add in major fluctuations for women like childbirth and menopause, and it can be a recipe for weight loss disaster.

Cortisol is a major stress hormone, and one of its effects is to trap fat around the midsection, which is one of the main weight loss problem areas. Cortisol production naturally increases as we age, and even more so in women than men (sorry, ladies!). This is a function of the adrenal glands, which also control the production of, you guessed it, adrenaline, and other metabolically-related stress hormones. Being able to control your stress levels will keep your adrenal glands from going into overdrive and producing too much cortisol.

To alleviate stress and keep tabs on your hormones to have better control of your weight goals, be in tune with your body. In the next section, we'll be talking about mindfulness and meditation, which can help you better recognize what your body and your brain are trying to tell you. If you are trying your best to stick to your weight loss plan and still find yourself stymied, it may be time to see a doctor and have your hormone levels checked. You may have an underlying lack or excess that is causing you to be unable to change your metabolism.

Finding Your Center With Mindfulness and Meditation

Getting caught up in the bustle of daily life and not knowing how to escape, calm down, and refocus your mind and body can be frustrating! That frustration can lead to even more stress, and then you're stuck in a vicious cycle. When life throws you a bad day, when you're feeling overwhelmed, or when you just need to find something in your life that relaxes and refocuses you, then meditation and mindfulness can become your best friends.

It's tough to make a major lifestyle change, and if you're working at losing weight while navigating today's crazy world, it can be even tougher. You're trying to adjust your schedule to include exercise, time to cook healthy meals or make smoothies, get enough rest, and still keep up with work, school, activities, and the kids! That probably makes you think you don't have time to cram in even more with meditation and mindfulness, but we promise you, you do. You don't have to devote a ton of time to these exercises, but the benefit you will reap will pay dividends.

Mindfulness and meditation can help you fight that old foe, stress eating. In the rest of the section, you'll find exercises and techniques that take just a few minutes or as long as you like, and you can use them to avoid reaching for the comfort food, get to sleep faster, and clear your mind when stress gets to be just a little too much. All good meditation and mindfulness techniques are founded in the ability to take good, cleansing breaths, so let's take a look at some breathing techniques to get you started.

The first breathing exercise is closely associated with yoga, but it has many different applications. Getting more oxygen to your brain is a great way to start calming down and thinking clearly, so when you feel stressed or foggy, try a few deep **yoga breaths**. Straighten your spine, and exhale all the air from your lungs. Now breathe in deeply through your nose, keeping your shoulders level and letting the air fill your lungs. You should feel your diaphragm expand downwards into your gut. Hold that breath for a three count, and slowly expel it all back out through your mouth. Repeat three or four times until you feel yourself relax. You may feel some tingling in your feet and hands as properly-oxygenated blood flows to your extremities.

The next breathing technique we'll go over is **box breathing**. This method is taught to military and police as a quick way to resolve immediate stress a regain focus. It is as straightforward as it sounds; you are going to breathe in a cycle of four parts, for a count of four. First, expel all the air from your lungs. Without breathing in, count to four. Now breathe in through your nose, also counting to four. Hold your breath, you guessed it, counting to four, and exhale through your mouth, counting to four. Repeat, of course, four times. It may take you a few tries to stop trying to instinctively breathe in immediately after inhaling, but you'll get the hang of it with practice.

The last breathing technique we'll cover here is **4-7-8 breathing**. The name of this method refers to the length of the count. First, you want to straighten your spine and exhale deeply, making sure your lungs are empty. Next, take a breath in through your nose, counting to four.

Hold that breath for a count of seven, and then exhale through your mouth for a count of eight. Repeat three or four times. Because you are exhaling longer than you are inhaling, be sure to be sitting the first few times you try this technique. You can become a little lightheaded until you get used to practicing it. This method clears and oxygenates your system, boosts your metabolism, and calms your heart rate.

Now that you know how to breathe, per se, let's take a look at some meditation and mindfulness techniques to put your breathing techniques to good use and move your stress relief in the right direction. First, we'll define the difference between meditation and mindfulness, because the two are often used interchangeably, and that isn't quite the case. While both meditation and mindfulness are meant to help you calm down and be able to focus, they aren't the same.

Mindfulness is based on the foundation of being present in the moment. This means clearing your mind of all other things and focusing on a single mental task or train of thought. It helps you remove stress and overstimulation from the emotional equation and find awareness. Mindfulness can take just a few moments or as long as you like, and is a useful tool for handling anxiety, stress, problem-solving, and sleeplessness.

Meditation is also used to alleviate stress, anxiety, and insomnia, but instead of directing you to focus on in-the-moment awareness, it can go one of two ways. Meditation can ask you to completely empty your mind and let go of everything you've been holding inside, or it can ask you to pinpoint focus on one idea or mantra that will help you to calm down or place all your energies in that mantra. The nice thing about mantras, and we'll get into them in-depth in a little while, is that they can be used throughout your daily life to evoke that feeling of focus and relaxation that you have when you are actively meditating. This can jolt you from a moment of stress and indecision into knowing exactly what you need to be doing.

Let's start with one of the most useful mindfulness exercises, one that takes moments and can save you from an all-out anxiety or panic attack. It's called the **5-4-3-2-1 grounding method**, and it's taught by mental health professionals worldwide to help people calm down and come back to their center at times of overwhelming stress. It's easy to remember, easy to do, and can be an emotional anchor.

When you feel yourself getting overwhelmed, or think you've got an anxiety or panic attack coming on, you can use 5-4-3-2-1 grounding to alleviate the immediate stress. First, take a couple of deep yoga breaths to start slowing your heart rate down. Then look around you and identify five things you can see- anything works, so it could be a pen, a desk, the carpet- just list them to yourself. Next, identify four things you could touch- the upholstery on your office chair, the drapes on the window- and imagine how they might feel. After that, identify three things you can hear- a colleague talking on the phone, the drone of the air conditioning, etc.- followed by two things you can smell, like a cup of coffee or a scented candle. The last step is to identify one thing you could taste. This can be silly or realistic- please don't actually go lick the window, for example.

When you've completed the exercise, you will feel much calmer. You've refocused your brain away from the stimuli that were causing you to go into a panic. A similar quick stress relief mindfulness exercise is the **3-3-3 method**. In this version, you will take a couple of yoga breaths; then you can identify three things you see, then three things you hear, and then consciously move three parts of your body (wiggle your toes, flex your hands, etc.). This is a short exercise you can do anywhere at any time to refocus your anxious energy.

The next mindfulness exercise we'll look at is one that you can use every day to remind yourself to be more present in your own life. When you have greater spatial and situational awareness, it makes you a better decision-maker- and if you are making or following a weight loss plan, one of the key elements of success is making smart food and exercise decisions. This mindfulness exercise should probably be called 'huh, I never noticed that!' but it's better known as **situational mindfulness**. Think about something you do every day. This could be your drive, ride, or walk to work or school, or a particular chore you do at home, like washing the dishes.

When you are completing your daily activity, challenge yourself to pay attention to your surroundings. If you ride the bus to work, try to count how many stop signs there are between your house and your office. If you're standing in front of the sink window washing dishes, challenge yourself to see how many birds are flying around your backyard. Choosing a challenge and sticking with it during your entire activity is a great way to learn to be more observant and more attuned to what's going on around you. When you practice this mindfulness exercise regularly, you'll find that problem-solving and decision-making start to become easier. This is because you've begun to open up new neural pathways to take in, sort, and process information more efficiently. Isn't the human brain an amazing thing?

When you've got time to sit and relax, there are a few mindfulness exercises you can do to further your journey to be calmer and making headway on your weight loss goal. The first is a **white light exercise**. Sitting comfortably, you should take a few deep breaths to clear your lungs. Next, imagine that there is a white light directly above your head. Now picture that little ball of light starting to expand and begin to envelop you, slowly, from the top of your head, down your arms and torso, down your legs and over your toes. Once your entire body is bathed in that imaginary white light, reverse the process. Make the light recede all the way back up your body, off the top of your head, and then slowly fade away. You will feel a tremendous sense of calm and clarity.

Another similar exercise is a **mind-body mindfulness** technique. Again, sitting or lying down comfortably, take a few cleansing breaths and think about your toes. Yes, really. Now slowly transition into thinking about your lower legs, your knees, your upper, legs, and so on, until you've gotten to your head and then down your arms to your fingers. You can move each body part slightly as you think about it to keep your focus. Think about how your toes feel against the carpet, or how your calves are achy after a long day of work. Concentrate on making a specific, conscious, relevant thought about every part of your body. This creates a sense of mind-body awareness that you can then reference when you are making decisions about changing your body through weight loss.

You can use the white light exercise and mind-body exercise to help you calm down and find focus to be able to think critically about other things that are going on in your life. When you begin to practice mindfulness regularly, you will find that you also begin to live a life of mindful intention. You will find yourself being more observant, less quick to jump to conclusions without enough information, and more confident in decisions that *do* need to be made with haste or without much warning. You'll find yourself being calmer, kinder, and sleeping better, and you will definitely find yourself making better, more informed food choices.

If you're having trouble sleeping, and the other exercises aren't providing the full relaxation you need to fall asleep faster, here's one last mindfulness technique to give you some calm, clarity, and peace at night. We've all heard the old wives' tale that counting sheep can help you get to sleep, and this exercise is based on the same premise, that the rhythm and order of numbers can be soothing. In this **countdown method**, you're going to get yourself nice and comfy and start at 100. Count slowly backward, being sure to think about each number- it's not a race. If you're really good about concentrating on numbers and not everything else that could be racing through your head, you'll never get to 'one'- you'll be asleep by the fifties!

Now that you've got a nice range of mindfulness exercises to consider, let's also take a look at meditation. Meditation, as previously discussed, is a conscious effort to either free your mind completely or focus solely on one idea. Instead of asking you to be more in tune with the world around you, like mindfulness, meditation asks you to be more in tune with your own thoughts and feelings. When some people think of meditation, they might think about ancient yogis sitting cross-legged and humming. While there are plenty of ancient yogis sitting cross-legged and humming, that's not all there is or can be to meditation.

You can meditate anywhere while wearing anything. You just have to be able to get into the right mindset, and if you like, you can set aside a particular time of day, like in the morning, before bed, or after work, to do a daily meditation and affirmation session. Creating a routine should be an important part of your weight-loss strategy, so adding planned meditation to help you relieve stress and help you focus on good decisions can be a great addition to your plan.

When you meditate, you should decide what you want to meditate on *before* you begin. That way, you won't be wasting precious meditation time on thinking about what you're supposed to be meditating about. Find a comfortable place to sit, and close your eyes. Take a few cleansing breaths and release the tension in your shoulders. Now, focus! Yes, it's easier said than done. This is why mantras are great. When you decide what you want to meditate on, you can create a short phrase or saying to remind you of what you're supposed to be thinking about.

For the purposes of sticking to your weight loss plan, you can try mantras that remind you of your goals. For example:

"Today, I will make good food choices."

"Today is a gift; I will use it wisely."

"Drink enough water. Eat smart foods."

You get the idea. These snippets are meant to keep your thinking on track and concentrate on your goals. Free your mind of all other thoughts and focus only on what you want to train your brain to do. If you meditate regularly on goals and actions relevant to your weight loss plan, you'll find that the things you are meditating on will become second nature, and you will be able to move onto other things to meditate about.

Learning to use meditation and mantras to remind yourself of important goals is a great way to retrain your brain to make better decisions that are based in calm introspection rather than in the heat of the moment. The best part about mantras is that you don't have to be in your meditative state to use them! They stick with you, so the next time free food pops up in the breakroom at work, you can look at the donuts and the veggie platter, and tell yourself, "Today, I will make good food choices," and feel confident in your decision to have the veggies, or treat yourself to a slowly-enjoyed half a donut.

Meditation goes beyond 'sitting around and chanting mantras,' too. You can use meditation to think about whatever you'd like, anything that's going to calm you and help you feel more centered. Perhaps you'd like to use your meditation time to think about somewhere that makes you happy. You can concentrate on picturing yourself laying on the beach listening to the gulls and the waves. If you meditate on your 'happy place' and it induces a sense of calm, the next time you're feeling overwhelmed, you can close your eyes and quickly picture your beach scene to quickly evoke that sense of calm.

Meditation is about knowing what will make you calm and focused and teaching your brain how to retrieve that sense of calm whenever you need it. By choosing to meditate on very specific things, you will make those things a permanent part of your neural pathways. It's a wonderful way to learn more about yourself, find your center, and be a better decision-maker when you need to make choices on the fly.

If you have a hard time getting into the groove of meditation and mindfulness techniques, there are a lot of wonderful books, audiobooks, guided audio and video exercises that you can download or subscribe to on your phone. These guided meditations will help you learn to practice on your own. If you have a tough time, don't be tough on yourself! Practice makes perfect when it comes to meditation and mindfulness, so just keep trying. If you find your mind wandering, gently guide it back to your exercise, and don't get frustrated. Frustration is counterproductive to the stress relief you are seeking. Be kind to yourself! Learning how to use meditation and mindfulness as a component of your weight loss plan is all a part of the journey.

Hypnotize Yourself

The use of mantras is almost akin to self-hypnosis, which is a great way to think about how you talk to yourself about making choices. In the movies, we see characters in deeply brainwashed states, activated into action mode by a keyword or phrase, turning the mild-mannered accountant next door into a covert operative. You've seen stage hypnotists convince people to be chickens by 'putting them to sleep' and snapping his fingers. While these are exaggerated versions of hypnosis, that's what using mantras can do for you. It activates your brain into making the designated choice attached to that mantra.

Using self-hypnosis through mantras is a great way to give yourself gentle reminders to follow through on the choice you've told yourself to make. There are other ways to nudge your psyche and do the things you've put into your plan. You can put your morning supplements next to your car keys, so you remember to take them on the way out the door. If you've never been a 'take my lunch to work' person, make it the night before when you finish dinner and put your keys in the fridge with the lunch bag, so you remember to grab them both. Take advantage of the alarm settings on your smartphone and create reminders for yourself for these types of things.

When you're trying to not only lose weight but create new habits for life, you'll need every little psychological trick you can find to help yourself along. Think about how you talk to yourself and how you can improve your inner monologue. Look at these two sentences:

- "I'm glad I went for a walk this morning, but I can't believe I let myself have a second helping of potatoes tonight, ugh!"

- "Well, I couldn't resist that extra spoon of potatoes tonight, but I at least I went for that walk this morning."

These say the same thing, but it's how you phrase yourself that matters. In both these sentences, you've recognized that eating the extra potatoes was not the best choice, but that taking a walk was a good decision. By ending on a positive note, you've recognized that you've made a small mistake and that you know you can do better, but you're not beating yourself up over your alleged potato crime. By using a positive inner monologue, you can change the way you think about yourself and your decisions.

Another thing you can do to hypnotize yourself into staying positive and continuing to make good decisions is to create affirmations. An affirmation is a short paragraph that you can read or recite every day to remind yourself of your purpose, your positivity, and your plan. You can think of an affirmation as a personal weight-loss mission statement. You want your affirmation to state your goal, your reason for it, and what you promise to do to achieve it while being kind to yourself. Here's an example:

I have committed myself to losing weight and learning to live a healthier lifestyle. I am doing this because I want to have more energy for myself and my family, avoid weight-related health concerns, and to raise my self-esteem and self-image. I am going to accomplish my goal by making smart food choices and getting more exercise, and I'm going to push myself to do this every day. I recognize that this will be hard work and that I may sometimes slip, but I will pick myself up, and it will all be worth it in the long run.

Another type of self-hypnosis you can do is visualization. This is a fun exercise in pushing your brain to imagine where you are and where you want to be. Sitting comfortably, close your eyes, and picture yourself how you are now. Then, picture yourself as you want to be. How can you get from Point A to Point B? Try taking an imaginary walk through your mind! You can picture yourself walking down a beautiful wooded path or through a quiet park. Think about the things you should pass and the things you should stop and observe to reach your goal of weight loss.

Practice, inside your head, walking past a street food cart and choosing not to stop, instead choosing to get an apple off the trees along your path. Look into the window of an imaginary home and decide if you should sit on the sofa or lay on the floor and do some yoga. The idea is to visualize yourself making good choices and walking a path to weight loss. Use your meditation brain to commit your imaginary world to memory. Whenever you have a difficult time making a decision, you can picture yourself as you imagine at your end goal and think about how making good choices got you there. It's a terrific motivator. In essence, you will think yourself slimmer. That's a great tool to have in your mental arsenal.

Now that we've taught you how to sit still, next we're going to teach you to get moving! In the next chapter, we are going to hike, walk, jog, dance, do yoga, lift weights...and never pay for a gym membership. We'll be talking about ways you can add physical activity into your weight loss plan, no matter your current weight or activity level. It's going to be fun; we promise! Let's take a look.

"The greatest weapon against stress is our ability to choose one thought over another."

- William James

Chapter 8: Get Up, Get Out, Get Moving: Exercise for Every Lifestyle

"Success is not final; failure is not fatal; it is the courage to continue that counts."

- Winston Churchill

According to the First Law of Motion, a body at rest stays at rest, and a body in motion stays in motion until acted upon by an outside force. When it comes to creating a weight loss plan and sticking with it, you're going to need to be the force that gets you moving. It can be an overwhelming undertaking to choose an exercise regimen and stick with it, but if you start off small, pick activities that are interesting and fun, and remember that something is always better than nothing, you can find ways to get up and get moving, stress-free. It can also be useful to find a friend to join you or find a group of people that are interested in the same activities. In this chapter, we're going to look at some things you can do at home and outside that won't cost you anything except your time and energy and will help you explore your capabilities and surpass your own expectations.

When you begin to exercise regularly, you will find not only a change in your physical fitness and stamina but also in your mental state. It can, quite literally, be addictive. Exercise releases endorphins, which make us feel great! Those endorphins can change the chemistry of the brain, and eventually, you'll begin to look forward to the feeling of calm and accomplishment that you get after a good workout. If you've ever heard the term 'runner's high,' it refers to the rush that distance runners get when their brain reaches maximum endorphin production. While the simple exercises that follow aren't likely to get you to that level of fitness euphoria, they will, simply put, make you feel better physically and emotionally.

You should talk you your health care provider about exercises that are safe for you to begin, especially if you have underlying health conditions. The point of exercising is to get moving and get healthy, but you want to make sure that you take part in activities that are going to be beneficial. Getting injured the first time you try something isn't exactly conducive to making you want to run back and try that exercise again. You also want to make sure that you're cleared to take part in any heavy cardio or weightlifting activities before you get started. The next sections are by no means comprehensive of all the different things you can do to get up and get active, but there's a nice variety of things you can do at home to get going and help you choose things you'd like to further explore. Let's get moving!

S-s-s-t-r-e-t-c-h!

Let's talk about stretching. It doesn't seem like true exercise, but it can stand alone as one to improve flexibility and circulation. It should also be used as a precursor for other activities to prevent injury. Warming up your muscles by stretching is a good way to slowly ease into adding other activities into your exercise regimen. Stretching also relieves stress, can alleviate edema and water retention, and to be honest, it just feels really good. Stretching can also burn up to 200 calories in an hour, so that's another good reason to try adding time for stretching to your daily routine.

Stretching is about pushing yourself every day to go just...a...little...bit...further. You should set your baseline before you begin any regular stretching regimen. Try to touch your toes without bending your knees. Can you do it? How far can you get your fingertips? Make a mental note, write it down, or have someone take a picture for you. Now try to stretch your arms up over your head. Can you hold your arms straight up, fingertips pointed to the sky, for thirty seconds, elbows straight? If not, time yourself and see how long you can last. Thirdly, sitting on the floor with your legs straight in front of you, lean forward and see if you can touch your forehead to your knees. Mark your baseline for that, too.

With three goals set- touching toes with straight knees, holding arms straight above head for thirty seconds, putting your forehead to your knees- you can begin a gentle stretching regimen. You only need to devote a few minutes to stretch every day, but the results can be astounding. You want to think about your body in the three segments- upper, core, and lower. Building flexibility and stamina in all three will help you be more successful at all your other chosen activities. That's why when someone has surgery to repair an injury, they go through physical therapy- the stretches learned there will build strength for all other activities.

Here's an assortment of stretches that you can try at home, with modifiers that can be used if you have mobility issues:

Lower Body- Stretching and strengthening your lower body is important because it will give you a strong base for all your other activities. You wouldn't set your stuff on a table with wobbly legs, so when you do your leg stretches, think about how you are improving your foundation for better balance and stability.

   - *Pancake stretch*: This seated stretch is simple and works and groin areas. Seated on the ground (or in a straight-backed chair), open your legs until you've formed as wide a 'v' as you can. Reaching above your head, take a deep breath, and bend yourself forward as far as possible. You want to reach your hands forward and lower your upper body as far as you can between your legs. Try to hold your position for 10 seconds, working your way towards a 30-second hold.

- *Quad stretch*: This standing stretch is for the long quadriceps muscles on the front of your thighs. Standing with your feet together and your spine straight, lift your left foot and grab it behind your back with your right hand. Try to hold for at least 10 seconds. You can modify this stretch by placing your free hand on a chair back for assistance with balance or by holding your foot in your same-side hand instead of the opposite hand. Once you've stretched your left leg, swap and stretch your right. Repeat 3 times on each leg.

- *Lunges*: This standing stretch keeps your hamstrings stretched and strong. Starting with your feet together, take one giant step forward and shift your weight from your back foot to your now-front foot. You can put your arms out to the side for balance or place a hand on the back of a chair to modify. Hold the lunge for at least 10 seconds, then bring your feet back together and switch feet. Repeat 3 times for each leg.

Core- Your lower back and your abdominal muscles will thank you for the stretches and strengthening! When your core gets stronger, you will experience less back pain, be able to lift and bend with more flexibility, and feel stronger and more fit overall.

- *Seated back twist*: This stretch opens up your lower back and oblique muscles for better core flexibility and less lower back stiffness. Sitting on the floor with your spine straight and your legs together out in front of you, bend your left leg at the knee and cross your legs, planting your left foot to the outside of your right knee. Now twist your upper body and give your left knee a 'hug" with your left arm while planting your right hand on the floor behind you. Hold for ten seconds, then switch legs. Repeat 3 times for each side. To modify this exercise, sit in a straight-backed chair, and cross your left leg over the right. Now twist to your right, and grasp the front corner of the chair seat with your left hand and the back of the chair with your right. Hold and repeat as above.

- *Spine bridge:* This stretch strengthens your abs and glutes for better core stability and stamina. Laying on the floor with your knees bent and your arms at your side, lift your hips and arch your back to lift your core towards the ceiling. Hold your lifted position for 10 seconds, gradually working your way to a target of a thirty-second hold. You want to have your body form a triangle from your feet to your hips to your shoulders on the floor. If you need to modify this exercise, you can bend your arms to give you leverage as you 'push' your core upwards.

- *Straight leg raise*: This exercise works your lower abdominal muscles for better overall core flexibility and strength. Sitting on the floor with your legs out in front of you, lean back and rest on your elbows. Now lift your right leg, toes pointed, as high as you can and hold it for 10 seconds. Lower your leg and do the same with your left leg. Lower your left leg and then raise both legs together and hold. Repeat three times. Modify this exercise by sitting in a straight back chair and holding the sides of the seat as you perform your leg raises. Work towards a thirty-second hold in each position.

Upper Body- Stretching and strengthening your upper body will make you feel refreshed, give you more muscle stamina when doing other exercises and activities, and give you better posture and less shoulder tightness.

- *Arm circles*: This stretch loosens your arm and shoulders and builds stamina. Standing with your feet shoulder-width apart, raise your arms out parallel to the floor, like a 'T.' Start moving your hands in small circles, gradually widening the circles until you are swinging your full arm in a sweeping motion. Reverse the direction and decrease the size of your circles until only your hands are moving again. If you need to modify this exercise, it can be done sitting down in a straight-backed chair. Make sure you keep your spine nice and straight like you're being suspended from an invisible thread atop your head.

- *Chest opener:* This stretch opens up your chest and rib cage, where the muscles are often tight from sitting at a computer at work and school. Standing facing a corner with your feet shoulder-width apart. Placing one forearm on each wall of the corner, lean in. You want your face to go into the corner as your shoulders and chest stretch back and out against the resistance of your arms. The farther you place your feet from the base of the walls, the deeper your stretch will be. This exercise should not need to be modified but can be done sitting down if necessary.

- *Biceps stretch:* This stretch lengthens and strengthens your bicep muscles of the upper arm. Standing with your feet shoulder-width apart, put your hands behind your back and lace your fingers together. Lift your hands as high as you can without separating them, and hold for 30 seconds. Work your way up towards holding for a full minute. Repeat 3 times. If you cannot stand during this exercise, it can be performed sitting down on the floor or on a stool.

There are stretching exercises designed to work out every muscle group in your body, and these are only just a handful of basic stretches to get you started. Work towards the flexibility goals we set at the beginning of this segment, and mark your milestones so you can see the difference for yourself. If a stretching regimen has you feeling good, and you want to expand your repertoire, there is a wealth of stretches and instructional photos and videos to be found online. Look for those from reputable websites and trainers.

Yes, You Can Do Yoga

The thought of yoga might be scary for some, but it's a worthwhile exercise that everyone can do regardless of fitness or flexibility levels. Yoga can build strength, flexibility, and stamina, but it also promotes patience and peace, all while burning up to 300-400 calories per hour. You also don't need much equipment for yoga, which is a terrific way to save money on a gym membership. You can get started with a simple foam mat and the internet- there are a ton of instructional videos and inexpensive streaming options to get you moving at home.

Here are some simple yoga exercises that you can do on your own, with modifiers that can be used if you have mobility issues:

- *Mountain pose*: This is a basic balance exercise that opens up the chest, stretches the spine, and gets your blood flowing in and out of your extremities. It also strengthens your legs and buttocks. It is a standing pose, so if you have balance concerns, you can modify it by keeping one hand on the back of a chair during the pose or by putting your back against a wall.

To complete the mountain pose, you should stand, spine straight, with your feet flat and hip-width apart (the better your balance becomes, the closer you can put your feet). Next, take a deep yoga breath and 'sink' your toes into the ground to anchor you. With your hands resting calmly at your sides, palms turned slightly out, take deep yoga breaths, feeling your shoulders blades stretch, and your chest open up. Keep your legs and back straight as you take several breaths and feel your body open up and become more relaxed.

- *Warrior I pose:* This next standing pose can also be modified by holding the back of a chair with one hand to maintain balance. This pose is similar to the lunges we talked about in the stretching section above, where you will be balancing your weight between your front and back foot to stretch your leg muscles. The arm movement added to this pose opens up the chest and the shoulders and improves circulation.

To complete the Warrior I pose, stand with your feet slightly apart. Taking a deep yoga breath, lift one foot and place it forward in a lunge position and exhale. Try to balance your weight evenly between both your feet. Taking another breath, raise your arms above your head as you inhale. You should end the pose with your arms extended straight above your shoulders, and fingers pointed to the sky. Inhale again and lower your arms back to your sides as you exhale, then bring your feet back to rest together to finish the complete move.

- Corpse pose: No modifications are needed for the corpse pose, as it is a still pose performed on the floor. To complete the corpse pose, lie flat on your back, feet slightly apart, hands at your sides, palms to the floor. Close your eyes and take a deep breath, letting your spine and ribs sink into the floor and feeling the tension go out of your shoulders and legs. Repeat until you've taken ten breaths, and sit up slowly when you're done to avoid lightheadedness.

- Downward dog: One of the most well-known yoga poses in the world is the downward dog, and it works to give you a great full-body stretch and opens up the rib cage and spine. To modify the downward dog, you will need a straight-backed chair placed against a wall, seat facing you.

To perform the downward dog, start on your hands and knees. Taking a deep breath in, rock backward, so you are sitting on your feet, then breathe out as you raise your hips and lean forward onto your hands. Draw your hips toward the ceiling as you form a triangle- head down, arms and legs straight, hips as the apex. Hold this pose for ten seconds, working your way toward a 30-second count. Be sure to breathe deeply as you lower yourself back to the mat. To modify, begin standing, feet hip-width apart, then bend forward and grasp the sides of the chair seat firmly. Lift your hips as high as you can toward the ceiling, and hold the pose. Even though you are not getting full arm extension to the floor, you should still feel your lower back and hamstrings stretch and loosen.

- *Tree pose:* The tree pose is a standing form that encourages good balance and steady breathing. To modify, you may use a chair back to place one hand on for balance, or you may place your lifted foot on your ankle rather than your knee.

To complete the tree pose, stand with your feet together, hands at your side. Taking a deep breath in, lift one foot and place the sole against the inside of the opposite knee (legs should look like the numeral 4), and raise your arms above your head, bringing your palms together directly above you. Hold for ten seconds, exhaling as you slowly bring your matched palms down to rest in front of your heart and place your foot firmly back to the floor.

- *Child's pose:* This pose is a classic resting pose to center your body and stretch your spine. It can be modified by using a chair, back against a wall to prevent sliding.

To perform the child's pose, kneel on the floor, weight resting on your backside. Taking a deep breath, lift yourself up and lean forward, resting your forearms on the floor and slowly sliding them forward until your head is touching the mat and your arms are straight. Hold for ten seconds, working your way toward a thirty-second hold. If you are modifying, kneel in front of your chair, and when you lean forward, grasp the seat of the chair on each side and rest your forehead on the edge of the seat. No matter how you do child's pose, you should feel your spine stretch and loosen, and your chest relax.

Tai Chi for Balance and Calm

Tai chi is an ancient Chinese martial art that focuses on centered, gentle movement, and balance. It can be a great introduction to movement for those who are interested in the martial arts but don't want to jump directly into more high-impact or combative styles. You may have seen tai chi practitioners in your local parks and admired the graceful movement of the poses. Here, we'll go through a basic tai chi sequence that you can do at home to improve balance and blood flow. While this is a very low-impact exercise, you should still warm up by lightly stretching before you begin.

The Warrior and the Scholar: This form will begin your tai chi movement sequence, and it is simple. Tai chi movements all tell a story, and this one is about a person who begins as if he is about to commit an act of violence (the warrior), but then thinks better of it and comes back to rest without striking (the scholar).

To perform the Warrior and the Scholar, stand with your feet slightly apart, as widely as you need to stay balanced. Relax your arms at your sides. Next, bring your feet together and bend your knees, and gently closed your right hand into a fist and place the palm of your left hand towards the ground. Slowly bring your left hand up to cover your right fist in front of your chest, then step forward with one foot. Uncover your fist, bring yourself back to a standing rest, and allow your hands to drop back to your sides.

From this resting position, transition into the next movement:

Golden Lion Shakes Its Mane: This form increases blood flow in the upper body and stretches out your spine. Its story is made obvious from the name- you will be mimicking the movement of a lion stretching and showing off its magnificent locks.

To complete Golden Lion Shakes Its Mane, move from a standing rest or sitting straight in a chair, to leaning forward. Move slowly until your trunk is parallel to the ground (or as far as you can comfortably go). When you've leaned forward as described, you are then going to twist your shoulders to one side, while moving your head in the same direction. Slowly bring yourself back to standing or sitting straight up, and repeat the movement, twisting in the opposite direction this time. Repeat this movement a total of ten times on each side, or as many repetitions as you are capable of.

From your resting position, you're going to move into another classic movement:

Brush the Knee: This form is a position that involves coordination between the upper and lower body. The story is one of a warrior cleaning his hands of violence as he finishes a battle.

To complete Brush the Knee from your rest at the end of the Golden Lion Shakes Its Mane, you are going to move into what is called the t-stance. Resting your hands lightly on your hips, put your feet together, and gently rest your left heel against your right ankle. Next, lift up your right arm, with your palm facing to the front.

Your left arm will be in front of you, palm facing the ground. You're going to step forward with your left leg and twist yourself slightly at the waist, pushing your right arm forward, and lowering your left arm. To finish the form, you'll next circle your arms back into a resting position and bring your feet back together.

To finish your tai chi sequence, you'll move into the following form:

Touch the Sky: This movement opens up the chest and rib cage. This tells the story of someone both showing vulnerability as they expose their torso and giving thanks to the sky for the ability to be peaceful.

From your resting stance at the completion of Brush the Knee, place your feet slightly apart and put your hands in front of you, palms up, with your fingertips facing each other. Next, you're going to take a deep breath, and slowly lift your hands over your head. Be sure to keep your arms slightly bent and loos. Hold your hands above your head, palms to the sky, and then exhale and bring your arms back down to rest. Repeat this movement five times.

It's recommended that tai chi be performed outdoors in nature. The reflective, calming effect of tai chi is also not to be ignored. Once you've learned the flow of the movements and regulated your breathing, you'll be able to appreciate the energy and story behind the forms. If you find that you love tai chi and the way it makes you feel, you can find a local group to join and learn more extensive forms and sequences. Tai chi is lovely proof that exercise doesn't need to be fast-paced or high-impact to have a positive effect on our bodies and minds.

Take a Hike! Walking for Fitness and Fun

One of the best and easiest exercises you can do is simply go out and take a walk. Taking a walk is free, involves an activity you've been able to do since you were a baby, and can be a stepping stone (no pun intended) to greater overall fitness. If you live in an urban or suburban area, you likely have sidewalks in your neighborhood, and if you live in a rural area without sidewalks, chances are good you don't have to worry about car traffic too much anyway.

Even if your roads aren't the best place to take a walk, there are always other options. You can see if the public is allowed to use the outdoor track facilities at your neighborhood school, or walk on your lunch break at work by taking a few laps around the building. You can also fit in a walk at a park before or after work. You don't have to be able to walk very far at first, but every little bit counts, and you can work your way up to longer distances over time. Try to start with a walk around the block, then two laps, and so on, until you can comfortably walk for about thirty minutes without needing to rest.

In our house, hiking is the name of the game. Even if you live in a city, you can find quality hiking within a short distance of your home. If you live in more suburban or rural areas, chances are good that you've got trails all around you. Hiking can be as easy or as difficult as you are willing to make it, so don't be afraid of the word! It might evoke visions of backpacking through the wilds, fighting the elements and warding off wild animals, but it doesn't have to be that adventurous!

By definition, hiking is the act of taking a walk through a natural setting. You don't have to climb a mountain to enjoy a good hike. Many communities have long, level trails such as rail trails (built on old railroad beds), and there are county, state, and national parks that offer hiking areas for all ability levels. When you take up hiking, you're opening yourself up to a whole new world of beautiful sights and natural habitats. Hiking can be more interesting than taking a sidewalk jaunt and can lead to other hobbies, like photography, birdwatching, rock climbing, and more. Another great thing about hiking is that you'll become so caught up in the nature around you, you'll soon not realize how far you've been walking. The best part? Every mile you walk earns you around 100 calories burned.

You can find places to hike in your region by doing a quick online search of nature areas. If you're planning on taking up walking and hiking, the best thing you can do for yourself is to get a good pair of shoes. While it may cost a little money in the short-term to get some quality footwear, it will be worth it in the long run not to have sore feet, knees, and hips, not to mention blisters. You should also get a pedometer or download a pedometer or tracker to your phone to keep tabs on your distances. If you've got a smartwatch or fitness tracker, even better! If you're not a fan of these technologies, you can always use a map to determine how far you've been walking. In the city, you can drive the route you normally walk to figure out the approximate distance, too.

Run Away! (Around the Block)

Maybe you'd like to set a bigger goal for movement and start running instead of walking or hiking. That's a great choice, too! Running is a great cardio workout and requires nothing more than determination and a good pair of sneakers to get started. While no one goes from zero to marathoner overnight, you can begin from nothing and work your way up to longer distances with practice and patience. Running can help you burn up to 350 calories an hour, which is a great return on an activity that only requires patience and shoes.

When you want to begin running, you're going to want to test out your endurance. That's great, but you don't want to hurt yourself by doing too much, too soon. Take the time to stretch before and after every run, and don't be afraid to rest during your running sessions. You can alternate running and walking while you're working out, and be sure to stay hydrated. You should also take any aches or pains seriously. Running can be impactful on the lower body and spine, so rest and care for any strains or swelling, and consult a doctor if they continue. If you can afford to do so, you should get fitted for good shoes and/or orthotics by a podiatrist. It will vastly improve your running mechanics if you've got the proper footwear.

There are also some terrific publications and websites out there devoted solely to running. You should check them out and get a good sense of how to develop running goals, how to treat runners' injuries, and how to deal with things like chafing (a real problem for distance runners), and where and how to join local running clubs to find new friends and a support system.

No Gym Necessary: Using Everyday Objects for Strength Training

Many people choose to purchase gym memberships because they are looking for access to free weights and strength training apparatus.

This is a great pursuit, but you've got weights hidden all over your home if you only know where to look. The advent of online training videos means that you can learn proper form and function right in the comfort of your home.

Some people avoid weight training because they think that the only purpose is to develop large muscle mass like a bodybuilder, but this is a well-worn myth. Weight training can be used to build lean, toned muscles by using smaller amounts of weight and performing more repetitions. You can also use weight training to increase your endurance, up your heart rate, and burn calories at an average of 200 an hour. Here are a few simple weight training exercises you can do at home with everyday objects:

Milk jugs: A gallon of milk (or the jug filled with water) weighs just over eight pounds when full. If eight pounds is too heavy for you to start, try half-gallons or don't fill the gallon jugs all the way. Similarly, a 72 oz jug of laundry detergent weighs about five pounds. These are useful objects because they have built-in handles, and you can use a jug to complete several home weight training exercises. Try these-

- Biceps curls; holding a full jug by the handle, lift the jug toward your shoulder, keeping your elbow still as you bend it and your forearm tight. Repeat ten times on each arm.

- Dips; holding a jug in each hand, keep your back straight. Bend your knees as if you were going to sit on a chair, then stand back up. Repeat the dip ten times.

- Lunges; similar to the dips, hold a jug in each hand and alternate lunging onto one foot, keeping your weight evenly balanced. Repeat lunges ten times each side.

- Pectoral curls; holding a jug in each hand, sit upright on a straight-backed chair. Lift the jugs out to your sides, arms parallel with the ground. Bring the jugs into your chest by bending your elbows. Touch the jugs to your sternum, and repeat ten times.

Backpacks: Backpacks make great workout gear because you can fill them with as much or as little weight as you like. Try using a backpack in these ways-

- Walking weight; to build strength and stamina, load your backpack evenly with the weight you want to carry. Being sure to wear the pack correctly, with both straps and snugly against your back, not resting on your buttocks. Take a walk with your pack on, and increase the weight gradually until you can comfortably carry fifty pounds for a mile.

- Kettlebell substitute; use your backpack straps to mimic the exercises done with a kettlebell. Stand with your legs spread widely and well-balanced with the bag on the floor between your feet. Bend down and pick up the bag, one strap in each hand. Lift the bag towards your chest by bending your elbows, not by moving your spine. Hold the bag at your chest for a ten count, and put it back down. Do a total of ten repetitions.

Here are some more ideas for strength training with everyday objects:

Paint cans: The handles on paint cans make them a perfect candidate for weight training at home. Grab a broom and two cans and make a farmer's yoke for carrying, dipping, and lunging with extra weight.

Books: Heavy textbooks make great weights. Keep one on your staircase and carry it up and down with you every time you make a trip between floors in your house. You can also use a textbook as a weight on your back when doing push-ups or to hold while doing sit-ups.

Sack o' taters: If you don't have any milk jugs, you can use a 5-pound bag of potatoes to complete your exercises. Try holding your bag of potatoes at your chest, then hoisting them straight up above your head to see how long you can maintain your lift. Just don't drop them on your head!

Child's jump rope: Well, you could use it to jump rope, but you can also use jump ropes, lengths of cotton clothesline, or towels as resistance bands to help you hold your form as you stretch and work out.

You can also use your own bodyweight for simple resistance exercises. For some people, getting onto the floor for things like push-ups and sit-ups can be difficult, but good news! If you've got a wall and a chair, you can modify these exercises to fit your ability levels and gain core and upper body strength. Here are some modified forms of common body-resistant exercises that you can try:

Seated crunches: Sitting on a straight-backed chair, grasp the sides of the seat, and straighten your spine as if being suspended by the top of your head. With your feet flat on the floor, tighten your lower abdominal muscles, drawing your feet off the floor, and bringing your knees toward your chest. Hold for a ten count and lower your feet back to the floor. Repeat a total of ten times. Don't worry if you can't lift your legs very far with just your abs. Resist the urge to use your legs to help. You will build up your abs over time and be able to draw your legs higher the stronger you get.

Standing push-ups: Stand facing a wall, with your feet shoulder-width apart. Place your hands flat on the wall at chest height, and lean in until your elbows are bent, and your chest touches the wall. Repeat a total of ten times. When you are comfortable with using your body weight in this position, move towards using the seat of a chair placed against a wall to do your push-ups. When you are comfortable with this position, move to doing modified push-ups on the floor, with your knees on the ground as you move your upper body. Finally, transition to a full standard push-up. Bonus points for doing all of these exercises while wearing a weighted backpack.

Wall squats: Regular squats are performed free of any props, but for those with knee or ankle issues, squats can be painful. To do this terrific quad and buttock exercise without too much distress, you can complete them with your back against a wall. Standing with your back straight and your feet hip-width apart, slide down the wall as if you were going to sit on a chair. The goal is to get to a 90* angle with your legs but go as far as you can. Hold for a ten count before sliding back up into a standing position. You can move to holding a chair back for balance and then transition into doing unassisted squats as you become stronger.

Fingertip sit-ups: Lay on the floor with your knees bent, feet on the floor, as if you were going to do a traditional sit-up. Instead of putting your hands to your ears or the back of your head, you're going to place your arms up over your head, laying them on the floor, palms up. Now, swing your arms up over your torso and touch your knees with your fingertips. This creates the momentum and torsion needed to contract your abdominal muscles. Repeat your fun swinging movement as many times as you can, aiming for reaching 25 repetitions as you build up your stamina.

These are just a few ways you can modify and work your way toward the more standard and advanced versions of these common and familiar bodyweight exercises. Try them, and you'll be surprised at just how much you can accomplish when you put your mind to it. As for using household items for weight training, have fun with it! Challenge your family to see who can come up with the most creative 'home gym' ideas, and then put them to use.

Dance Your Butt Off

Who doesn't love music? Even the grumpiest among us are prone to a toe-tap when they hear a great beat. No matter your culture or your taste in music, you can get up and get moving to burn calories with dance. The great thing about today's technology is that we have music at our fingertips at all times. We can stream it from several different smartphone applications, listen on our computers, and tune into our cable and satellite providers' music choice channels.

You don't have to be a trained dancer to dance your weight away; all you have to do is feel the beat. Turn on some music, shove the furniture out of the way, and have an impromptu dance party with your kids. Dance in your bedroom, your backyard, the kitchen while you're cooking dinner. You can burn up to 400 calories with just a half-hour of dancing, so give it a try! You'll be happier and healthier in no time, just by letting loose a little. Music lifts our spirits and dancing melts away calories and releases endorphins, so there's nothing to lose except weight.

There are also some great workout routines based on dance, including ballet and tap. These include some basic stretching and footwork designed to get you moving and learn flexibility and balance. If you've always wanted to be a ballerina, or at least mimic their lean muscle mass, then you might look into a hybrid barre workout regimen. These incorporate some of the things we've already discussed, including stretching and endurance. Tap-inspired workouts are more of an aerobic endeavor and are great for adding fun cardio to your routine.

You can dance on your own, try a style-based workout class or video, or even take a ballroom dancing class with your partner. You'd be surprised at how much fun a foxtrot or waltz can be when you are learning it with someone you love and losing weight at the same time. Latin dance is also a great cardio and endurance training activity. However you choose to get your dancing done, have fun with it- it's definitely okay to dance your butt off!

More Ideas for Getting Fit

Exercise can be anything that you want it to be. The idea that gyms and clubs are the only ways to get fit is outdated. If you want to try something, try it! You can try road cycling or mountain biking. Go swimming regularly, or take up martial arts! Cancel your landscape contractor and buy a push mower, or take up gardening. Raking, digging, bending, and weeding can burn a few hundred calories an hour. Even standing up at work instead of sitting down can add to your daily calorie burn. Live near a lake? Find a deal on a secondhand kayak and paddle your calories away.

For the more adventurous, consider taking a kickboxing class, or trying out a rock-climbing wall. Both of these activities have become very popular in the last decade, and there are facilities available in most urban and suburban markets. Cross-fit is another type of training that is seeing surging popularity because it offers a lot of variation and caters to all ability levels. If you're into walking and hiking and want to add to your experiences, try geocaching or metal detecting to add a bit of treasure hunting to your outings. Join a local adult rec league for a sport you enjoy, or sign up to coach youth sports and share your expertise while working out with the kids.

To get your whole family involved in getting fit, set up family challenges like obstacle courses or sidewalk chalk mazes. When you engage in exercise as a family activity, not only are you finding better fitness, but you are modeling it for your children. Try finding parent and child workout videos, or hold footraces in your backyard. If you are showing your kids healthy behaviors, they will want to emulate those behaviors. Don't expect your first-grader to consistently choose a salad over a bag of chips, but teach them that it's okay to eat in moderation, and that exercise is important to keep them growing big and strong.

If you like racquet sports, you can learn to play or get active with tennis, badminton (easy to set up in your backyard!), racquetball, or pickleball, which if you're not familiar, is played on a modified tennis court and has been likened to playing life-sized ping-pong. Pickleball is easier on the joints than traditional tennis and is becoming tremendously popular. Check around your area for racquet clubs to get involved, even if you just treat yourself to a day pass occasionally. Even pub sports like darts, billiards, and bowling can get you up and get you active; ask around town to see if there are any leagues that you can join.

The fun thing about finding ways to get active is, well, finding new ways to get active. You can go to a local farm and go on a trail ride, or volunteer to be on the clean-up crew at your local park. The only limit to being active is your imagination. There are so many ways to get in motion, so be creative! Challenge yourself to walk to the next tree, to the next rock, or around the block one more. Run or swim one more lap, and be proud of all your accomplishments. When you set exercise goals and achieve them, it's an amazing feeling.

Be Social and Find Support

Exercising on your own can be boring and frustrating. That's one reason that group classes are so popular at gyms. But if you're trying to save money on a gym membership, how can you find a support system to keep you moving and motivated? It's so important to find workout friends who can offer encouragement and advice, and provide company when you're exercising outside of your home.

You can always ask your family and friends to work out with you, which can be a great way to get everyone moving and feeling fit. But what if you live alone or don't have many friends living nearby? You can find groups online almost everywhere for almost any type of fitness endeavor. There are running clubs and walking groups dotted through almost every community.

Many areas have cycling organizations and hiking clubs, too. The internet makes it easy to find people with similar interests in your area.

The boost of motivation that comes from having people to both exercise with you and have your back when you need support is immeasurable. It's proven that people who have a support system lose more weight than people who do not, so get involved! You'll find new friends, you'll get your workouts done, and you'll feel better physically and emotionally. Please don't be ashamed to share your goals with others- no matter what physical state you are starting from. If you want to take up running, advice from people who are veteran runners will be invaluable. Everyone starts somewhere! Don't be afraid to ask for help.

The key to sticking to a fitness plan is to find something you really enjoy so that it won't feel like a chore to do it. In the next chapter, we'll take a look at bringing all the parts of your weight loss goals into a manageable plan with notes, mantras, and schedules that you can follow to achieve success.

"Don't let what you cannot do interfere with what you can do."

- John Wooden

Chapter 9: A Plan, A Path, A Promise, A New You!

"By recording your dreams and goals on paper, you set in motion the process of becoming the person you most want to be. Put your future in good hands- your own."

- Mark Victor Hansen

Let's think about what it means to be 'successful.' How do people succeed in school, at work, in their hobbies? While there are instances where an individual might fall into accidental success, the majority of the time, success is earned through hard work and careful planning. Here, we'll begin tying together everything we've discussed throughout the book and talking about how to write down your plan, set your short-term and long-term goals, and getting started.

Dream It Up and Write It Down

Way back at the beginning of the book, we briefly went over the concept of realistic goal-setting. One of the best things you can do for yourself is to dream big and think small. That's not to say that you start by believing that you won't achieve the big dream. No, what we mean is that you should break your big dream down into small chunks to make each step seem more manageable and keep you motivated.

You should have by now gotten yourself a sturdy notebook or journal, or a good fitness application for your computer or smartphone. You want to have a written or digital record of your goals and your progress. There are some fantastic free applications that track food, exercise, sleep, and other metrics, and if you have a wearable fitness tracker, you can sync the applications to keep track of all your movement and food.

When you track your food, sleep, and exercise, you can begin to see patterns in your behavior and appetite, which can help you be smarter about your choices. For instance, if you see that you tend to grab more convenience food on days after a bad night's sleep, or feel empowered by having a smoothie and a salad after a good workout, then you can track what you need to do to make smarter choices. Behavior patterns are what will teach you about how you are progressing and when you can declare that a habit has been made or broken.

Setting goals and being realistic as what you can achieve within certain timeframes is also crucial to being successful. It's great to say that you want to lose 50 lbs, but if you don't have a plan or milestones, how will you reach your goal? Keeping in mind that average, healthy weight loss is one to two pounds per week, how are you going to time out your benchmarks? A good place to start on a 50 lb weight loss goal is to set it out over the course of a year, which is just over 52 weeks. You may, of course, lose more weight than a pound a week, but to be realistic and kind to yourself, this is a very manageable goal.

Take your calendar or notebook and mark out the half-year mark, then the quarter-year marks. Don't worry about pounds per week yet, we'll get there in a minute. You've now broken your goals down into 12.5 lbs lost every 13 weeks. That's amazing! You're setting yourself up to lose less than a pound per week. Anything over that is an overachievement, isn't that fantastic? Now that you've figured out how to break your goals down into small pieces, you can mark the dates in your calendar and set goals in your weight loss journal or tracking application.

With your goals set, let's talk specifically about how you're going to go about reaching them. In the chapters that preceded this one, we talked about learning to read food labels and being a smarter consumer. We also looked at meal replacements and supplements, smoothies, and shakes, and getting started with some exercises and fitness inspiration. To achieve a great change, you've got to set that change in motion. What's your plan?

While nobody likes to feel deprived, it can be difficult to make a huge change in diet and not feel that some sacrifices have been made. If you ate three candy bars and drank 2 liters of cola every day for the last ten years, then you're not going to immediately take to eating salad and drinking smoothies without feeling a little bit grumpy. It's okay to ease into a healthier diet. You can switch from sugary sodas to diet colas, and then onto iced teas and coffees, and then plain water.

Write down what you want to achieve and what you're willing and able to do to get there. Think about the dietary changes you want to make, the foods you like to eat (or would like to learn how to eat), and the things you should cut back on or eliminate. Using these lists, you can begin to form your meal planning lists. You can also begin to choose any supplements you think you'd like to try and if you think you'd like to try the intermittent fasting method.

Once you've done all your food-related contemplation, think about exercise. What strikes your fancy? Do you want to try hiking or running, or are you more of a casual dancer and gardener? Getting your exercise in should be fun, safe, and interesting, so think about what you'd like to do and what kind of time you can carve into your schedule for these activities. Yes, we know that adding anything into your already busy life can be difficult, but it is possible, and you're going to find a way, we promise.

Think about the time you spend now in passive recreation, watching TV, playing on the computer or game console, and just wasting time on your smartphone. If you spent ten, fifteen, twenty minutes fewer each day in those pursuits, you could find the time to add in some yoga or stretching exercises. You can take one or two days a week to get up just a little earlier to take a walk before work and take an evening away from the television to learn a new sport or activity. It's possible to find the time, but you have to want to do it. That's another reason that finding a social group can be so uplifting and important- you cannot deny the motivation from others is really helpful in getting you up and moving.

The third component of your weight loss plan will be the stress-relief factor. How will you use mindfulness and meditation to help you lower your stress levels and get better sleep to aid you in your goals? It doesn't take much time, but it does take an effort to be thoughtfully mindful each day. You can set aside a little time before bed to meditate, or do a mindfulness exercise before you get out of bed each day. There's no telling what life will throw your way every day, but if you are mindful, use your breathing and quick-fix grounding methods to deal will sudden stress, and approach each day as a new opportunity to do the right thing, then you will find yourself feeling calmer and more optimistic as a result.

Writing things down makes them feel more real, and once you've written down the three components of your plan- food, exercise, and stress relief- it's time to combine them into the big picture. You can create a roadmap and timeline to get yourself from Point A (your current weight and lifestyle) to Point B (your goal weight and lifestyle). Choose a start date, and set appointments to see any necessary health professionals, especially if you've got any underlying conditions. Then use what you've learned, use the things you want to achieve, and use your motivation to make these changes to write down a realistic plan to reach your goals.

Words to Live By: Creating Mantras to Keep You Moving

Okay- you've got a plan, and that's fantastic! Now, how are you going to remind yourself to stick to it every day? Mantras are a great way to keep yourself motivated when life creeps in. In a perfect world, you'd get up, do some meditation, have a breakfast smoothie, and practice mindfulness on your way to work. At work, there would be no stress; you'd make a smart choice for lunch, come home, and walk a couple of miles before having a healthy dinner and relaxing to wind down to get a good night's sleep.

-Record scratch- That's not how life works in today's fast-paced society. That's why mantras work so well, to remind us of our goals even when life is shoving stress and obstacles in our faces. Come up with a few little sayings that you can repeat to yourself or put on sticky notes on your desk or workspace. Some examples might be to remind yourself to 'take the stairs' when you need to move around your school or office building. Another might be 'wouldn't you rather have water?' when you start to reach for a sugary soda.

Engraining these little phrases into your brain is easy. The human brain loves repetition; that's how we learn. Think about the repetition you see in a small child's storybook. The reason that children love these books and eventually learn to read from them is repetition, which creates the neural pathways that commit things to memory. Muscle memory is the same way. When you repeat a motion often enough that it becomes second nature, it's difficult to then stop that motion. This is how habits are formed and broken, and you want to break away from the habit of being unhealthy and into the habit of making good choices.

In a way, this is a form of the self-hypnosis we talked about earlier. You want to train your brain to respond to certain stimuli (your mantras) with a certain behavior (making a good lifestyle choice). This sort of conditioning will eventually lead to you making the choices on your own without needing the mantras. That's when you'll know you've achieved a permanent lifestyle change. Then, it's time to make new mantras to get to your next set of goals. Little by little, you will make good choice after good choice, until you've reached the personal overhaul you are seeking.

Oh No, Now What? Adjusting Your Goals When Life Happens

Sometimes, life happens when we least expect it. What will you do if something major comes along, and you feel like your life has been derailed? Unexpected career developments, family issues, illness, and abrupt changes in our personal lives can have us feel like we are floundering and struggling just to survive. What weight loss plan? We were on a weight loss plan? And there it goes out of the window as stress creeps in and takes over. Sometimes, stress skips the window, kicks down the door, and makes itself at home. Now what?

You pick yourself up and dust yourself off, that's what happens now. It is okay to grieve the loss of friendship, the death of a family member, the sudden relocation, or even disappearance of your job. Humans are both blessed and burdened with the ability to feel emotion very deeply, and our emotional health has a definitive effect on our physical health. It's tough! But the best thing you can do for yourself is to try. Try every day to stick to your plan, because it will give you something to feel in control of.

When life is just the worst, you can still be your best. Find the strength to get up and go for a walk. Make yourself a small, healthy meal to keep your metabolism going. Allow your body to rest and renew at night. Worrying doesn't change anything, but action can. Give yourself the tools it needs to complete those necessary actions by eating, sleeping, and moving as much as you are able. If you find that you need professional mental health guidance, please don't hesitate to seek it out. It is a sign of strength to be able to say, "I can't do this on my own."

If your life situation has changed to the point that you need to rethink your goals, that's okay, too. Much in the same way you wrote your original plan, you can rewrite your story. Maybe you broke your leg, and you can't go hiking for a couple of months. That's unfortunate, but not the end of the world. You can work on upper body strength and stretching. You can burn off some calories crutching around the block. Where there is a will, there is always a way.

Maybe you need to relocate unexpectedly for work or personal reasons. Think about the people that make up your support system. Can the leader of your running club refer you to the leader of a similar club in your new city? Will there be a supermarket in your new neighborhood that fits your dietary and budget needs? Thinking critically about what you need to maintain your current plan will help you figure out what you need to do to revamp your plan in a new place.

The point us, as important as it is to write down your plan and your goals, it's equally important to remember that a pencil has an eraser for a reason. You can change your goals, your methods, and your focus. While it's recommended that you stick with your first plan until you can determine if it's effective, sometimes that just isn't possible. If you need to make a rapid change, then you need to do what's right for you.

What if it isn't a rapid change? What if something truly just isn't working, despite no vast, unexpected changes in your life circumstances? If you have made a solid plan, you've gotten underway, and you're confident that you've been trying your best, but you still aren't seeing any changes in your weight or energy levels, the problem may not lie in your efforts. You should consider seeing your doctor if you're 'doing everything right' with no results. You may have a previously-undiagnosed health condition, likely something endocrine like a thyroid or blood sugar concern. If you can address these concerns, then you can get back on your way on your weight loss journey.

Another reason you may decide that you need to adjust your plan is if you hit what's known as a weight loss plateau. You may find that when you first get started, you are losing weight at a steady clip, and then things seem to level off, leaving you wondering what you're doing wrong. The answer is probably nothing, but as you lose weight, your metabolism is changing, and your nutritional, caloric, and exercise needs may be changing as well. Try adding more cardio to your routine, getting more sleep, and adjusting your calorie intake for your new weight. By switching things up, you'll jumpstart your body again. When you first start out, you will burn more calories because the heavier you are, the harder your body has to work to do so. As you slim down and become more fit, you won't burn as many calories per workout session, and you'll need to adjust your caloric intake to continue to lose weight.

If you are resolved to create, work with, adjust, and readjust your weight loss plan as life happens, you will see more success than someone who is unwilling or unable to adapt as needed. Be firm in your belief in yourself and your belief that no matter how weird or awful life can seem, it will get better. Then go out there and make it better for yourself. You can do it, you've already come this far, and you've got what it takes to get to the finish line, leaving stress, fear, and anxiety in the dust.

Eyes on the Prize: New Milestones, New You

Did you take a before picture when you started your weight loss journey? Did you write down your starting weight on the first day of your plan? Are you planning on writing down your weight and take photos as you reach your benchmarks? What we're trying to tell you is that you should.

Remember when you were little or when your kids were little, and someone who hadn't seen you in a while exclaimed about 'how big' everyone had gotten? When you don't see a child for a while, you can see the change in them immediately, but chances are good that the parents don't notice because they see their children every day. The same is true when you are working your way through a weight loss plan and major lifestyle change. You may look in the mirror each morning and not see a difference. This can be discouraging. But if you take photos periodically, you will see yourself evolve as you accomplish each new goal.

It's great to meet your benchmarks along the way, and you should be excited about all your victories. Give yourself an incentive to hit your goals, and you should write these incentives down to make sure you keep your promises to yourself. This could be something like taking a day off to go to the beach or treating yourself to a new book, video game, or hobby item that you've been eyeing for a while. This is also a great way to hold yourself accountable for your goals. It's part of the personal responsibility that you must take as part of undergoing your lifestyle change. No one but you can be in charge of the adjustments you are making, and that's a tremendously powerful position to be in.

Aside from the physical change of losing weight, think about the mental and emotional impact your new lifestyle will have. You'll feel better and have more energy, sure; but you will also be able to see yourself in a whole new light. You can take pride in your accomplishments, and you'll raise your self-esteem and self-image. When you feel more confident, you portray yourself with more confidence to the outside world. That sense of self can be more invaluable than anything else you gain or lose during your weight loss journey.

*"Whether you think you can or think you can't,
you're right."*

- Henry Ford

Chapter 10: Keeping the Journey Alive

"Believe and act as if it were impossible to fail."

- Charles F. Kettering

You've done it! You set a goal, came up with a plan, stuck to it, and hit your weight loss target. Now what? Staying motivated to maintain your new lifestyle can be hard. You can think, "Oh, I've lost X pounds, I can eat whatever I want now!" Before you know it, you've gained back some weight, you're angry with yourself, and you need to start all over again. That doesn't sound like a fun scenario. So how do we ensure that all your hard work doesn't go to waste? You need to solidify that your weight loss plan wasn't just temporary and is, in fact, a true, permanent change in lifestyle.

Maintaining the New You

Maintenance is a boring word, isn't it? It has a negative connotation of infinite work. Yes, maintenance means an ongoing, recurrent task for the purpose of keeping something in its current state. But maintenance can also mean preservation and continuity, and those are important words to focus on. You've worked so hard to get to where you want to be, so why would you not want to do everything you can to preserve and continue your new-found fitness?

Throughout the entire book, we talked about ways to make your weight loss plan less of a diet and more of a lifestyle change. If you've done everything according to your plan, then you should have seen results beyond the numbers on the scale. We discussed how being a label reader, and smart shopper would become second nature. We looked at how mantras become reality and how setting new ones means you will constantly be setting up your brain to learn new things. That's the true goal of this book, not to teach you how to diet, but to teach you how to live a purposeful, healthy lifestyle.

Once the scale hits the number you've been aiming for, it can be all to easy to step back and say, "I'm done." Don't give in to the temptation to do that. Reward yourself, sure, but reflect on your journey and realize that it will be easier to maintain than it would be to start from square one. Keep on creating new mantras and setting new fitness goals. Explore cooking different cuisines and trying new recipes for smoothies and shakes. Your maintenance will only be boring and difficult if you make it boring and difficult.

Find new workouts and exercise routines to keep things interesting. You can look for new trails to hike or bike, or go to a trial class at your gym. No one wants to do things that don't hold our attention; it goes against human nature. But if you've spent this much time and energy into changing your lifestyle, you certainly aren't going to want to backslide. Look for other instructional activities to supplement your 'new you,' too. You could take a gardening class or cooking lessons to learn new ways to connect yourself to your food.

If you've achieved your goal of creating a true lifestyle change, then maintenance won't even be necessary, because this is your new, healthy life and you will continue to make good choices without it feeling like work or maintenance at all. Yes, there will be days when it might seem easier to slip back into old habits. Life is going to throw curveballs at you, and you're going to want to grab a sack of drive-through cheeseburgers and wallow on the couch for the evening. But if you can find the courage to talk yourself out of your grease-laden pity party and into a long walk and a healthy dinner, then you know you've truly made core changes to the way you live.

Be Forgiving, But Don't Forget

So what happens if you do get the cheeseburgers and have a wallow? It's not the end of the world, we promise. Sometimes, the best thing we can do for ourselves is to forgive. We have to remember that we're human, and therefore, not perfect. Sometimes taking care of our mental health is more important than having a salad for dinner. The answers aren't always black and white, unfortunately. Is it better to work out when you're feeling sick to not break your routine, or take a few days to rest and get over your cold? These are things you will have to figure out along the way, but you should always make these choices with kindness toward yourself.

If one of the things you are struggling with is your relationship with food, which of course, we addressed a few times throughout the book, then kindness is key. If you understand why you relate to food the way you do, it's easier to identify why and when you're having a moment of uncertainty. Take these moments as a chance to reflect on why you're feeling that way and why you've embarked on a weight loss plan. When you're in a foul mood and standing in front of the refrigerator, remind yourself that eating a giant piece of cake isn't the answer.

Food is not meant to be a filler for anything else lacking in your life, and tell yourself that the immediate feeling of comfort from the cake isn't worth the guilt you may feel later. Walk away from the fridge and go do something else to work out your negativity. Go for a walk, play with your kids, watch something ridiculous on TV for half an hour. Then go back and cut yourself a small piece of cake. You've resisted the temptation to eat an unreasonable portion borne out of stress. Good job! The cake will taste better for having been a thoughtful rather than rash decision.

Using Your New-Found Discipline

If you've been disciplined enough to create, follow, and succeed at a weight loss plan, just think about how else you can apply these skills? Maybe you've been thinking about a career change, going back to school, or taking up a new hobby. You can use the skills you've learned to lose weight to succeed in these endeavors, too. In this book, you were given a ton of skills, even if you aren't aware of it. You learned:

- how to identify a problem and discern its root cause

- how to use calendars and lists to set and achieve short-term and long-term goals

- how to effect personal change through a change in activities

- how to use mindfulness to be more in tune with the world

- how to use meditation to be more in tune with yourself

- how to plan meals and be a savvy shopper

- how to read and break down product labels

- how to think critically about a set of options and make good choices

These skills, as applied to weight loss, can be applied to other facets of your life. You can use your new-found planning skills to brainstorm, equip, start, and complete any new project you put your mind to. Being able to use meditation and mindfulness will serve you well in every aspect because you will be calmer, well-rested, and clear-headed whenever you need to make a major decision. Your new shopping skills are going to be useful, too. Use your knowledge to make good choices whenever you are shopping, especially for big-ticket items. You'll be so glad you learned how to read labels.

Look Ahead, Not at Your Behind

Once you've met your weight loss goals, you can be so proud of yourself for your accomplishments! What are you going to do next? Setting new goals, fitness or otherwise, is a great idea. Like we just discussed, you've got the tools now to make and keep positive change a major part of your life. Look to the future and begin to set new milestones for yourself. You could become a weight loss mentor or coach, and help others take a journey similar to yours by teaching your skills to those who need them. You can expand your fitness goals to try competitive distance walking or running, or join an adult sports team. You've opened up a world of possibilities for yourself, simply by making and sticking to a life-changing choice.

The future is as bright as you want it to be, so think big and don't look back. When you look in the mirror, see your accomplishments, not your flaws. You're amazing, and you should believe that. While you should never forget where you came from, you should know that you've come so far and that matters. What matters more than what you see in the mirror is what you feel on the inside. Use your light to continue to improve your life and the life of others around you, and don't ever forget to be proud of yourself!

"At any given moment, you have the power to say: This is not how the story is going to end."

- Christine Mason Miller

Conclusion

Thank you so much for taking the time to read *Best Diet Products*, and we hope you learned a lot about yourself, your relationship with food and exercise, and how to create a new, healthier lifestyle for yourself. We covered a lot of information in these ten chapters, and you can use this book as a reference to refresh yourself anything you need a boost or want a reminder about any of our topics. Before we say good-bye, for now, let's have a brief recap of everything we discussed in the book.

In Chapter 1, we talked about being able to make the choice to lose weight and defining relationships with food. For some people, weight loss can be a life-saving change, but without understanding why it's necessary or where the extra weight stemmed from, it's impossible to be able to craft a manageable plan. You wouldn't renovate a house that's on a sinking foundation without first fixing the foundation, and that's what we want you to be able to do- fix the foundation so that all the other hard work isn't wasted. In this chapter, we also talked about how food, like other things, can be addictive, but seeing as you can't quit food, you will need to find ways to be a smarter eater, even if that means outsmarting yourself.

Moving on to Chapter 2, we started looking at nutritional and dietary supplements and how they can fit into a well-rounded weight loss plan. These products are meant to help you navigate the waters of lifestyle change, and should be used only with the intent to compliment your other efforts. There is no cure-all weight loss pill, but with the help of your health care provider, pharmacist, or specialist, you can find a regimen that works for you, even if it's just a good multi-vitamin to help you get your nutrition on track. Supplements for losing weight and building muscle should always be used according to package labels and proper dosing, and if you have any questions, you should ask a doctor or pharmacist for advice before taking anything.

Chapter 3 was our smoothie and shake chapter, yum! Replacing meals with delicious, nutritious drinks is a fabulous way to feel full without a ton of calories. It's also a great method for adding fruits and vegetables to your diet if you aren't a big fan of eating them- which is okay because some people have sensory issues with the texture of vegetables. That doesn't mean it's not still important to get the nutrients these foods offer, and putting the foods into a blender and making them into a refreshing cold drink is a good alternative. If the texture is still an issue, run your smoothies or shakes through a fine sieve to remove any particles before drinking.

In Chapter 4, we talked about intermittent fasting and defining the times you eat, rather than what you eat, as a viable factor in weight loss. While this isn't a method for cramming in as many calories as you can during a given day, this is a good way to train your metabolism to know when to expect fuel and when to burn calories. It can also help you get better rest- no more spicy food at midnight- and have more sustained energy throughout the day.

Chapter 5 was all about the hidden things we should be looking for in our food, and how to moderate them in our diets. Caffeine and alcohol, sugars, and fats are all lurking, waiting to throw us off course as we pursue our goals. It's important to know how our body processes the things we consume so that we can make the best choices for ourselves. The key takeaway is to remember that the more processed the food is before it enters our system, the less work our body will have to do to break it down, meaning it won't burn as many calories during digestion and absorption.

Chapter 6 was a long one, but chock full of information, and you're probably still trying to take it all in, sorry! Reading labels, recognizing proper portion sizes, and learning how to plan, shop, and prepare healthy meals is so crucial to any weight loss plan. There is so much data on one little food label, and when you are label-literate, you can make informed decisions about everything you consume. Look out for the hidden things we talked about in Chapter 5, choose items with well-balanced nutrition, and learn to have fun in the kitchen. It's okay to fail, burn things, and set off the smoke detector every once in a while- just keep learning, and you'll be amazed at how far your new skills can take you.

In Chapter 7, we talked about stress and the effects that it can have on stalling weight loss. Being able to manage stress through mindfulness and meditation can alleviate sleep problems, help regulate metabolism, and give us the peace of mind we need to focus on our goals. While you won't always be able to avoid stress, when you incorporate these mental exercises into your daily life, you will be much better equipped to handle it.

Chapter 8 was our exercise chapter, and it should have given you tons of inspiration for finding ways to work out without needing to head to a gym. While we don't discourage gym memberships and the great equipment and instruction you can find there, it's often a hurdle for people who cannot afford a membership to be able to get fit. You can ask your friends and family to give you gift certificates to your favorite fitness businesses when asked what you'd like as a birthday or holiday gift or take a part-time job at your gym to earn a discount off your membership. We just want everyone to know that with or without a gym membership, you can safely work out and have fun.

In Chapter 9, we finally started to pull everything together and talked about the importance of writing down your goals, setting your mantras, and being able to adjust both on the fly and when you know things aren't working. When you chronicle your journey, either through pen and paper or a digital application, you're not only recording your weight and your dreams; you are recording the true, real hard work that you've put into your plan. When you look back, you'll be so amazed at how far you've come, and you can be rightfully proud of your accomplishments.

To finish up the book, Chapter 10 talked about being the custodian of your newfound lifestyle. We discussed how to think about maintenance not as a chore, but as a labor of love for your new self, and how to forgive yourself for any backsliding without forgetting how to keep up the hard work. We are our own worst critics, so please remember to extend yourself the same kindness you would extend others and use any slip-ups as a learning opportunity, not a chance at self-flagellation. We wrapped up by talking about how to use the discipline you learned losing weight to make other major life decisions, and set new goals without looking back with any regrets.

So, we've come to the end of our time together. Thanks again, so much, for choosing to read *Best Diet Products*. We wish you all the best as you take what you've learned and head off into the world of weight loss. Good luck with finding your path to a new, healthy lifestyle, and don't forget to check back in when you need a refresher. Remember the three components of your plan- food, exercise, stress management, and you'll be just fine! We'll leave you with one last bit of inspiration for your journey:

"Great things are done by a series of small things brought together."

- Vincent Van Gogh